617.412   Kessler, Seymour.
KES
          Heart bypass.

$22.95

DATE			

HEART
BYPASS

Heart Bypass

. . . .

How to Prepare Your Mind, Your Emotions, and Your Self for a Successful Outcome

. . . .

Seymour Kessler, Ph.D.

St. Martin's Press ✖ New York

Design by Basha Zapatka

Illustrations copyright © 1995 by Durell Godfrey

Library of Congress Cataloging-in-Publication Data

Kessler, Seymour.
  Heart bypass : how to prepare your mind, your emotions, and your self for a successful outcome / Seymour Kessler.
      p.   cm.
  ISBN 0-312-11820-1
  1. Coronary artery bypass—Psychological aspects. 2. Coronary artery bypass—Popular works. I. Title
RD598.35.C67K47   1995
617.4'12'0019—dc20   94-46269
                                                         CIP

First Edition: April 1995

10   9   8   7   6   5   4   3   2   1

This book is dedicated to
the next generation:
my grandchildren,
Chaya, Avi, and Penina

CONTENTS

. . . .

FOREWORD

. . . .

Bypass surgery is an affair of the heart. It taxes one's physical, emotional, and social resources. It is an unwelcome reminder of the threat of death, physical decline, and discomfort. Yet, for all these reasons, it can represent a new lease on life, an opportunity to live differently, reevaluate life priorities, change relationships, and improve health maintenance routines. In order to emerge from this threat with some of these positive results, you have to take the threat seriously, but not let it take you over. That is what Dr. Kessler offers in this book: a means of understanding and working through the complex and difficult process of undergoing coronary artery bypass surgery. He describes the heart problems that lead to the surgery and provides practical guidelines for preparing for surgery. He provides information and tells how to obtain more—about your surgeon and hospital and the choices involved in the surgery. But obtaining information is only one part of the process of preparation. It is equally important to access, express, and learn from your own emotional reactions to the procedure. They should be expected, and giving them expression can help you prepare for the challenges ahead. Dr. Kessler suggests a variety of techniques that can be useful in anticipating and therefore mastering the stresses involved. He and his wife, Dr. Hilda Kessler, also a psychologist, describe in a very personal way his experience of going through bypass surgery. Reading this chapter, you will learn that you are not alone, that many of your own reactions or those of loved ones are universal. They suggest not weakness, but the fact that you are coming to terms with a difficult situation. Dr. Kessler also provides useful chapters on life after surgery, facilitating recovery, changing health habits, managing anger and other strong emotions, and developing life goals. Family members can be enormously helpful in facilitating recovery, and suggestions are made for helping a loved one who has had surgery and for sorting out its impact on your own life.

Alas, a book like this is all too necessary. Cardiovascular diseases are the leading cause of death in most of the Western world. In 1991, between 40 and 46 percent of all deaths in the United States, Canada, England, and Wales were attributed to heart disease. It has been estimated that 6.3 million Americans suffer from heart disease, and that this year alone 1.5 million will have a heart attack. Among these, about one third will die. In 1991, 407,000 coronary bypass procedures were performed, at a total cost of some $18 billion. Almost half of these procedures were performed on people under the age of 65; three quarters were performed on men. Despite the fact that the public is more aware of the risk factors for heart disease—such as smoking, high serum cholesterol levels, and inactivity—and despite the fact that this awareness has led to behavioral change, heart disease is still the major killer. Coronary artery bypass surgery remains a widely used treatment modality, but is rarely a "cure" for heart disease. It merely moderates the symptoms. The need for coronary bypass surgery should be seen as a wake-up call to change the care and feeding of one's body, rather than a solution to the problem. Nonetheless, one can live a full and effective life, even with serious heart disease, as this book illustrates. Indeed, while facing the realities, this book provides a sense of optimism and encouragement about how to make the most of a bad situation, feel in charge of the process of treatment, examine alternatives, and get on with life.

Do such approaches add anything to life, either emotionally or physically? A number of studies have shown that management of emotion (especially anger) and social support can positively affect people with heart disease, and may even improve their chances of survival. Stanford psychologist Carl Thoresen showed that heart attack patients who went to support groups designed to help them deal with stressful emotions, especially anger, had lower rates of subsequent heart attack than those who received routine medical care. Physician Ralph Horwitz of Yale found that heart patients who adhered well to a drug regimen had lower rates of heart attack, even if the drug was an inactive substance, a placebo. Cardiologist Dean Ornish of San Francisco showed that heart attack patients who met in weekly support groups, learned meditation, and followed a strict vegetarian diet showed actual reversal of heart disease, with widening rather than further narrowing of their coronary arteries. Similarly, our research group at Stanford has found that women with advanced breast cancer who meet in weekly support groups not only feel less anxious and depressed, but also live an average of eighteen months longer than control patients given routine care. Thus there is mounting evidence that the way we cope with illness is an important aspect of its treatment, and may influence the body as well as the mind.

When President Franklin Delano Roosevelt said, "The only thing we have to fear is fear itself," he was only partially right. There were indeed other things to fear, but he touched a nerve by emphasizing the part of the threat we could recognize and deal with. Fear, anxiety, sadness, and other emotions are not the enemy, they are means by which we take a threat seriously and move beyond it. If you or a loved one is facing bypass surgery, let this book help you master the threat: take it to heart.

Dr. David Spiegel, M.D.
Department of Psychiatry
Stanford University School of Medicine

December 28, 1994

PREFACE

. . . .

In nearly twenty years of practicing clinical psychology, I have worked with many individuals and couples who needed to make important decisions about or preparations for major surgery and other medical procedures. Frequently my work consists of steering clients toward sources of information, then helping them make sense out of that information, providing a sounding board for talking through and evaluating various options, helping them find courage to face known and unknown terrors, and last, but not least, helping them find meaning in their experience. Although I have not always been successful, I do know that I have helped many persons deal with their personal ordeal, and I take an enormous satisfaction in this knowledge.

In June 1990, however, *I* became the patient. The diagnosis was coronary artery disease (CAD), and bypass surgery was strongly advised. Following my own advice to others, I turned to the current literature and other sources to obtain up-to-date information, guidance, reassurance, and solace. I found several books, most of them written by physicians, that were invaluable in describing the technical aspects of the bypass procedure, but I was surprised to find how little was available that might help a person prepare psychologically for the surgery and for its possible impact and aftermath. Furthermore, what was available tended to provide a grim, glum picture of what could be expected. Although many patients experienced an improvement of their physical symptoms, psychologically the surgery was often portrayed as a disaster. Depression and long-term emotional crippling were the outcomes most often predicted. Hardly reassuring or comforting!

As clinical psychologists, my wife, Hilda, and I refused to accept this transmitted "wisdom" about bypass surgery. Our individual professional experiences told us that in most cases, when the patient had actively prepared for the surgery both physically and psychologically, healing, recuperation, and raised self-esteem were promoted and generally occurred. The mental attitude toward forthcoming surgery is one of the central factors promoting positive surgical outcomes. Substantial research in health psychology supports this viewpoint.

Our personal and clinical experiences also told us that when the broader life issues raised by bypass surgery were confronted rather than avoided, when the surgery was understood as a question of how one lived his or her life rather than simply as a medical problem, important positive, health-affirming life changes became possible.

Like any other major life event or crisis, bypass surgery has the potential for loss or for gain. On one hand, it may leave the person impoverished and defeated or, on the other, enriched and enhanced. It may close the person off from discovery of his or her essential self or it may open the person's eyes and heart to the discovery of unanticipated inner treasures. The outcome, we believe, is largely under the person's volitional control. One can choose and, with active efforts, can bring about the growth and pride that comes from the sense of having transformed one's life and mastered illness and fear.

In our clinical and personal experiences as well as in the experiences of the nearly forty individuals we interviewed in preparing this book, we found many instances of individuals who saw bypass surgery as an opportunity to initiate important life changes. These were often attempts to master and prevail over their physical and psychological limitations and handicaps, to renew commitments to life and health, and to find the kind of meaning in their situation that would transform setback to achievement, adversity to triumph, loss to gain.

Cardiac crippling, depression, bereavement, and the other phenomena often associated with bypass surgery are not inevitable outcomes of the surgery. In fact, we strongly believe that much of the so-called crippling described in the literature may be the result of inadequate preparation for the surgery and of other psychosocial problems, including iatrogenic ones, those induced by the medical system itself, rather than of the surgery per se.

This book evolved from our professional and personal experiences, and fills a gap in the information available about coronary bypass surgery. We hope that it will help prospective patients and their relatives and friends obtain a more balanced perspective of what to expect, and will help them prepare for surgery in a way that is likely to promote a positive outcome in both the short and the long term.

This book deals with some of the major issues bypass patients and their families are likely to encounter before, during, and after the surgery. I have attempted to distill and describe some of the practical techniques I and others have found to be effective in dealing with these issues, emotional and otherwise.

Coronary bypass surgery affects not just the patient but everyone in the family. It requires and demands changes in the thinking and behaving of nearly everyone around the patient. Spouses are particularly impacted by their mate's surgery and often years after the surgery they may still be reverberating from the events around the surgery and dealing with the emotional impact. Friends too are affected by the need for bypass surgery, and if their responses are made out of concern combined with a sense of helplessness, they may not always be constructive.

This book is written with four groups of individuals in mind. First is the person either contemplating bypass surgery or preparing for it. In particular, I wish to address the layperson who wants to take responsibility for his or her own health and health decisions and who wishes to minimize the potential traumatic impact of bypass surgery.

Second, this book is intended for spouses (or significant others) of bypass patients, the individuals who, aside from the latter, will probably be most affected by the outcome of such surgery. Spouses can play an important role both in helping the patient prepare for surgery and in fostering their recuperation afterward. This book addresses some of the fears and anxieties spouses commonly experience and provides guidance to help them deal with the practical and emotional aspects of bypass surgery.

Third, the book is written for the relatives and friends of individuals contemplating or scheduled for bypass surgery. Since relatives and friends may be affected profoundly by the fact that the individual is having bypass surgery, they too need to make their own preparations and to understand how their actions and words might promote or inhibit healing in the patient. Relatives and friends also play an important role in the patient's life after surgery. Not infrequently, out of a lack of experience, one does not know how to deal effectively with the patient and his or her spouse. This book offers some insights on how the patient and spouse might be feeling and what their needs might be. In addition, when the patient has had no opportunity to prepare for the surgery, friends and relatives might play an important role afterward in helping him or her face and deal with the life issues bypass surgery raises.

Finally, the book is intended for physicians and other professionals who would like to further their understanding of the inner experience of the patient and his or her family and to help these individuals prepare more effectively for bypass surgery and the healing process.

My wife, Hilda Kessler, Ph.D., helped me write the chapters "Heart Bypass: A Personal Experience" and "A Spouse's Perspective," and I wish to acknowledge, with love and gratitude, her assistance at every stage of preparing this book.

My wife and I would like to take this opportunity to thank the many bypass graduates and their significant others who shared their experiences and insights with us. We are also indebted to our friends and relatives for their support and encouragement. I wish to thank the following physicians who helped us on our personal journey and encouraged us to write this book: Drs. John Edelen, Ron Elson, Don Fischer, Marty Klughaupt, J. Scott Rankin, Gregory Robertson, Philip Schild, John Swartzberg, and Daniel Ullyot. Mr. Tom Greenwood, R.N., made several useful suggestions, for which I am grateful. Also, I would especially thank Gina Maccoby for all her efforts on my behalf and Barbara Anderson for her masterful editing.

HEART
BYPASS

INTRODUCTION

. . . .

WhEN in the late spring of 1990 I was told that I had to
have coronary bypass surgery, I turned to the current literature
to refresh my knowledge about the procedure, its risks and benefits, and for encouragement. Although I had helped others prepare for such surgery, I was just as vulnerable, frightened, and
human as they were. I wanted to be as informed and prepared as
possible, so off I went to my nearest medical library to "hit" the
books and journals.

I found several good books, most of them written by professionals, that discussed the bypass procedure, but their focus was
on the technical aspects rather than on the inner experience of
the surgery. Because my wife, Hilda, and I are psychologists, the
inner meaning of bypass surgery was as vital and important to us
as its physical meaning. I was particularly troubled by the fact
that much of the literature tended to emphasize the adverse,
crippling side of the surgery rather than the physical and psychological benefits or gains that might be achieved for the person.

As I discussed the forthcoming surgery with physicians, I
found that they almost invariably tended to reinforce the down
side of things, the infirming consequences of the surgery rather
than its revitalizing potential. For example, almost every

physician I spoke to emphasized how virtually all individuals become depressed following bypass surgery as if this was a proven scientific truth. It is not.

Although I appreciated, given the current litigious climate in which medical practice occurs, that physicians feel obliged to inform their patients about the drawbacks as well as the benefits of a medical procedure, the way it tended to be discussed left the impression that the net losses of bypass surgery outweighed the gains and rewards. To a large extent these conversations planted the seed of this book in my mind.

Each year in the United States, about 400,000 coronary bypass procedures are done. Of these, 73 percent were performed on men. Nearly half of bypass operations are performed on people under 65 years of age. Individuals requiring such surgery generally fall into two groups, one consisting of persons in the throes of having or having had a heart attack, and the other consisting of persons who choose (or are advised to choose) the procedure on an elective basis either to prevent a heart attack in the relatively near future or to relieve severe angina symptoms that are unresponsive to other modes of treatment. The persons in the first group have little or no choice about the procedure since their lives are immediately threatened. Those in the latter group are often fortunate enough to have time to think about and plan for the surgery.

The perception of choice and personal control appears to have a decisive impact not only on how someone prepares for surgery but also on how he or she responds to it afterward—medically and psychologically. On the whole, persons choosing bypass surgery on an elective basis tend to respond to the surgery in a more adaptive way than persons who require the procedure on an emergency basis. I found, for example, that "elective" patients tended to recuperate faster than patients whose surgery was "imposed" on them, and had fewer difficulties, postsurgery, in effecting and maintaining health-promoting lifestyle changes than the nonelective group. However, even when bypass surgery was required on an emergency basis, persons who believed that they had control over their fate tended to behave differently both before and after surgery than those who took a more passive approach. Some individuals who had heart attacks, for example, used the short interval of time between the attack and the surgery to great advantage to prepare psychologically and emotionally for the surgery and for life afterward, and many had a remarkably rapid recovery and positive adaptations. Even though they were in some distress, they continued to perceive that they had control over their medical fate and over their lives.

TAKING AN ACTIVE STANCE

There are two ways to approach bypass surgery: passively and actively. The two approaches have different psychological meanings for the individual and his or her family, and in many instances foster different psychological outcomes.

Taking an active approach means being involved in as many steps of the decision-making process as possible. This includes making the decision to have the surgery, as well as deciding where and when it will be done and by whom. Being active also means positioning oneself psychologically for a rapid, effective recovery and thorough healing. In contrast, passivity means letting others make choices for us and accepting that whatever happens in and as a result of the surgery is outside one's control.

In his book *Taking Charge of Your Medical Fate* (New York: Random House, 1988), Lawrence Horowitz, M.D., former staff director of the U.S. Senate Subcommittee on Health, writes:

All physicians want to do right by their patients. The problem is that many times there are different views of what's right. And although a surgeon can change his view over time, and even change his approach to particular diseases as the medical evidence changes, you, as the patient undergoing surgery, never get a second chance. Taking charge is about maximizing the chances for success the first time.

Taking charge means being active in promoting your self-interests. Taking charge means assuming responsibility for your efforts to heal and recuperate. Thus, recuperation and later health are not dependent on chance events or passive processes, but rather on the efforts of the patient in achieving and restoring health. The normal healing processes of the body and the psychological and behavioral efforts are joined in partnership to accomplish a common goal.

An active approach toward health has long been recognized as having enormous power. In his book *Healing from Within: Psychological Techniques to Help the Mind Heal the Body* (New York: Simon & Schuster, 1986), Dr. Dennis T. Jaffe writes:

> Our power to prevent and heal illness is far greater than most of us realize. . . . If you are ill, it is essential . . . to become an active participant in the therapeutic process. . . . While it may be reassuring to imagine that medical technology will eventually deliver you from illness, modern medicine . . . cannot guarantee good health unless you work in conjunction with your physician. . . . [T]he key to enduring health often lies in your own behavior.

An active psychological stance is also likely to lead to changes in lifestyle that will prevent recurrence of the behavior and problems that led you to bypass surgery in the first place.

THE PRICE OF PASSIVITY

A passive approach is seductive; it's often the path of least resistance. In his book *The Mirage of Health: Utopias, Progress, and Biological Change* (New Brunswick, NJ: Rutgers University Press, 1987), Dr. Rene Dubos writes:

> To ward off disease or recover health, men as a rule find it easier to depend on healers than to attempt the more difficult task of living wisely.

In taking a passive approach the person gives up a part of his or her autonomy. "Make the decision for me. You are so much more knowledgeable than I. I will do whatever you say." This is the message of a person who wishes to abrogate responsibility for his or her health. In the early decades of the twentieth century, it was expected that the patient would play a passive role in regard to the physician. But times have changed and medical decision-making has become too complex to leave to physicians alone.

Passivity has many consequences. A passive approach promotes ideas of victimization—"They are doing this to me"—and deprivation—"I have suffered." In turn, these ideas promote the wish for reparations, compensations, and rewards later on. These "rewards" often take the form of eating those occasional creamy desserts, fried eggs, thickly buttered croissants, and dripping strips of bacon, and behaving in other ways that are antithetical to health and that tend to promote coronary artery disease. It is no wonder that many individuals who have already had bypass operations need further bypass surgery later on.

Over and over again, psychologists find that individuals who felt that surgery was externally imposed on them and that they had no choice about it, tended to have greater difficulties, physically and mentally, in the postsurgical period. In addition, when such lifestyle changes as giving up smoking, changing one's diet, exercising regularly, etc., were called for after the surgery, these changes were more difficult to sustain among such individuals than among persons who believed they had personal control over their medical fate and health.

Are psychological activity and surgery compatible ideas? Yes. True, at some point the patient needs to become passive so that surgery can proceed, but this is different from being passive about passivity. One can actively choose passivity as a response to surgical necessity. By doing so the patient retains responsibility for the choice. Psychologically, the patient has remained active in protecting and furthering his or her interests. This is in contrast to the helplessness involved in not choosing and in not deciding for oneself, an attitude that does little to promote optimum healing and recovery. Individuals who respond in an active way take responsibility for their health, whereas persons who choose a more passive approach give up responsibility for their health to others.

ABOUT THIS BOOK

This book encourages an active approach to one's own health and health decisions. In the chapters that follow, the reader will find not only useful information about bypass surgery but also a perspective about the surgery and about health in general that emphasizes taking responsibility for the maintenance of one's health.

Chapter 1 provides an overview of the essential anatomy and physiology of the human circulatory system and the biomedical facts concerning coronary artery disease (CAD) and its treatment are reviewed. It is important that some of the basic facts be understood, if for no other reason than to demystify the body and its physiological processes, as well as the medical attempts to deal with CAD. Also, a better understanding of the process of CAD may help the individual understand what must be done in the long run to maintain or improve the health of his or her coronary arteries.

Chapters 2 and 3 explore the best ways to prepare for bypass surgery, practically and psychologically. Chapter 2 outlines some of the practical issues the prospective patient (and his or her spouse) may want to consider. These include suggestions on how to choose a surgeon and a hospital, and how to get one's affairs in order before the surgery. At the end of the chapter is a suggested to-do list as well as a list of questions to ask the candidates when choosing a surgeon.

Chapter 3 considers some of the major psychological issues involved in preparing for the surgery, the immediate postsurgical period, and life afterward. There is no one way to prepare for major surgery. Any one or a combination of various procedures might be used with success. The main point is that some method or methods should be attempted rather than leaving such things to chance. The preparatory work advocated is designed to increase one's awareness and help one obtain greater control over one's life and life habits—in short, an active approach.

Preparing for the surgery is a way of preparing for a life of health afterward. Thus, the individual enters the surgical theater with confidence about survival and healing and with a sense of mastery and optimism about the future. At the end of Chapter 3, some exercises are suggested that do not require enormous psychological expertise and that might be used either by yourself or together with your spouse or significant other.

In Chapter 4, my wife, Hilda, and I describe our separate experiences with bypass surgery during the week of my hospitalization. Our perceptions and concerns proved to be markedly different. Hilda, in particular, will deal with the potential impact the patient's bypass surgery might have on other members of the immediate family.

Chapter 5 considers the problems of the postsurgical period, paying particular attention to the initiation of the lifestyle changes bypass surgery often demands of the patient and his or her significant other. Whatever gains one obtains from the surgery require active efforts to maintain. This may mean major changes in what one eats and drinks, and the adoption of exercise routines and other disciplined habits that may completely transform how one lives one's life. The message of bypass surgery is that it is time to live a healthy life.

Chapter 6 further explores the impact of the surgery on the patient's spouse and family. In our clinical experiences, Hilda and I have found that the needs and emotions of the spouse are frequently neglected by physicians. Although they are not subjected directly to the surgeon's scalpel, their distress, sometimes trauma, is certainly as great as that of the patient. Moreover, given the situation, spouses frequently feel that they have no justification for expressing or voicing their fears, concerns, and pain. This, in turn, may lead to behavior that is in the interests of neither spouse nor patient. In some instances, years after the surgery spouses were still reacting to and reverberating from the event. Their view of and confidence in the patient as a partner (and, at times, as a viable human being) was shaken and sometimes changed dramatically.

Finally, Chapter 7 tries to make sense of the whole experience and to find some transcendental meaning in it. Bypass surgery does not cure coronary artery disease. All it does is give the person a second chance at cleaning up his or her act. Once the surgery is over, one is faced with a choice about how to live out the rest of one's life. One can pretend one is healed and return to the patterns of living that are virtually guaranteed to re-create the atherosclerotic conditions that necessitated surgery in the first place. Or, one has the option of choosing to live, in the fullest sense of the word, with a commitment to health and awareness. This is the path I recommend.

ONE

. . . .

THE MEDICAL FACTS YOU
NEED TO KNOW ABOUT HEART
BYPASS SURGERY

This chapter reviews the basic details concerning the circulatory system and coronary artery disease (CAD), and describes some of the current treatments for CAD, including medication, balloon angioplasty, and coronary bypass surgery.

THE CIRCULATORY SYSTEM

The individual cells of the body require nourishment in order to function. The circulatory system transports this nourishment—oxygen and nutrients—to the cells, and carries away the waste products produced as a byproduct of metabolism—the chemical processes through which the body produces energy and assimilates new material—within the cells. The major waste product is carbon dioxide.

The components of the circulatory system are the heart and the blood vessels—the *arteries, veins,* and *capillaries.* The heart is the central pumping station of the body. The blood vessels are like a dynamic plumbing system. The arteries carry oxygen-rich blood away from the heart. The main arteries branch off into smaller and smaller ones until they become capillaries, tiny blood vessels that penetrate the organs of the body. It is through the capillary walls that oxygen is given up as nourishment to the cells. Other capillaries remove the carbon dioxide from the cells. These capillaries join together to form larger vessels known as veins, which carry the oxygen-depleted, carbon dioxide–laden blood back to the heart.

The Heart of the Matter

The heart is a saclike muscular structure, roughly the size of an adult fist, located behind the sternum (breastbone), near the midline of the body. Internally, the heart is divided into four chambers. The two upper chambers, called *atria* (*atrium,* singular), receive blood from the veins. The two lower chambers, called *ventricles,* pump the blood through the arteries to the various organs of the body. See Figure 1.

The right atrium receives oxygen-depleted, carbon dioxide–laden blood from two major systemic veins, the *superior and inferior vena cava.* When the right atrium contracts, the blood passes downward through a valve, the tricuspid valve, to the right ventricle. The valve keeps the blood from flowing back into the right atrium when the ventricle contracts.

The ventricles function as the major pumping stations of the heart. The right ventricle pumps the oxygen-depleted, carbon dioxide–laden blood through the pulmonary artery to the two lungs, where the blood gives up the carbon dioxide and replenishes its oxygen supply. From the lungs, the oxygenated blood returns by way of the pulmonary veins to the left atrium. From there, it passes through the mitral valve to the left ventricle. The left ventricle then pumps the oxygenated blood through the *aorta,* the major artery of the body. Arterial branches coming off the aorta distribute the blood to the major organs of

INSIDE THE HEART

Figure 1

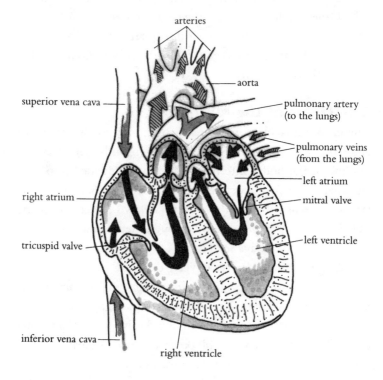

Carried by the superior and inferior vena cava, carbon dioxide-laden blood enters the heart at the right atrium and travels through the tricuspid valve to the right ventricle. It is pumped to the lungs to be replenished with oxygen. Oxygenated blood returns to the left atrium and passes through the mitral valve to the left ventricle. It is pumped throughout the body through the arteries that branch off the aorta.

the body, the branches becoming smaller and smaller as they enter the organs, finally becoming capillaries.

Among the first arteries branching off the aorta are the main *right and left coronary arteries,* which go directly to the muscular walls of the heart, called the *myocardium.* See Figure 2. The unimpeded delivery of oxygen to the heart muscle is essential to support its pumping activity, which in turn supports the enormous variety of activities of the body under normal conditions as well as under stress and exertion.

The Coronary Arteries

The main coronary arteries are about a quarter of an inch in diameter at the point at which they branch off from the aorta. From there they run along the surface of the heart, branching into vessels of increasingly smaller diameter that dive deeper into the heart tissue. The right coronary artery runs down the outer surface of the right side of the heart and usually provides blood flow to the lower wall of the left ventricle, sending out branches that sink into the muscular tissue.

The main left coronary artery, as it leaves the aorta, divides almost immediately into two branches, the *left anterior descending artery* and the *circumflex artery.* The left anterior descending artery runs down the front surface of the heart just to the left of midline and sends branches to the left ventricular muscle. The circumflex artery curves to the left and goes to the back side of the heart. It also sends out branches to the left ventricle. In the presence of developing CAD, small blood vessels called *collaterals* may begin to develop to provide blood flow to the heart muscle from adjacent arteries. However, these alternate pathways may not be sufficient to prevent a heart attack in cases where a sudden occlusion, or clogging, of a coronary artery occurs.

If you took a cross-section of an artery you would find that it

CORONARY ARTERIES **Figure 2**

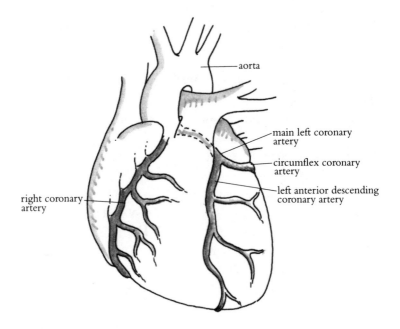

The main right and left coronary arteries branch off the aorta and provide blood to the myocardium, the muscular walls of the heart.

is not just a pipe through which the blood is transmitted (see Figure 3). In cross-section, an artery looks somewhat like a tube surrounded by a layer of smooth muscle that itself is surrounded by a layer of fibrous connective tissue. The innermost layer of the artery is lined with a thin layer of flat cells called *endothelial cells* that allow the blood to pass through the vessel with a minimum of friction. (If the friction is low, so are the chances of damaging a blood cell; a damaged blood cell could lead to clot formation.) Surrounding the endothelial cells is the muscular layer and, finally, there is an outer layer of connective tissue holding it all together.

HEART DISEASE, CORONARY ARTERY DISEASE (CAD), AND HEART ATTACKS

The term heart disease covers a group of disorders involving the structure and/or functioning of the heart and the coronary arteries. Infections, chronic high blood pressure, and other factors may affect the effective functioning of the heart. For example, a streptococcal infection of the throat, if not treated, may lead to the development of rheumatic heart disease, in which the valves of the heart are damaged. Some individuals are born with congenital heart problems as, for example, mitral stenosis, a disorder of the valve that separates the left atrium and left ventricle. When the muscles of the left ventricle contract and push blood through the aorta, the mitral valve keeps the blood from being forced back up into the atrium. A mitral valve that loses its elasticity may allow blood to regurgitate into the left atrium, thus decreasing the effectiveness of the left ventricle's contraction. Open heart surgery may be needed to repair or replace the faulty

PROGRESS OF CORONARY ARTERY DISEASE   Figure 3

endothelial cells

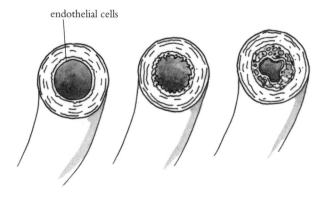

The leftmost figure shows a normal, healthy coronary artery. The inner wall is smooth and blood flows easily. The middle figure shows roughening of the endothelial layer of cells. This is caused by injury to the artery wall, sometimes due to smoking or high blood pressure. The rightmost figure shows the accumulation of plaque and the thickening and swelling of the artery wall associated with coronary artery disease (CAD). This is the condition in which coronary arteries are blocked or narrowed due to fatty buildup, known as atherosclerosis.

valve. Another type of heart disease occurs when the muscles of a ventricle are damaged because of a heart attack. This too compromises the capacity of the ventricle to carry out its pumping function and has serious consequences for the person's health and ability to function.

A heart attack occurs when the blood flow to the heart is slowed or stopped for long enough that the heart muscle, or myocardium, is damaged, usually permanently. The medical term for a heart attack is *myocardial infarction,* or MI for short. An MI is caused by a clogged or blocked coronary artery, resulting from fatty buildup (atherosclerosis), a blood clot (coronary thrombosis), or spasm. Some 40 percent of the half a million people who have heart attacks in the United States each year do not survive them.

The condition in which the coronary arteries are narrowed or blocked due to fatty buildup is called coronary artery disease, or CAD. How this fatty buildup, or atherosclerosis, occurs is explained on pages 23–24. CAD is the primary cause of heart attacks. The coronary arteries bring oxygen-rich blood to the heart muscle. Without this continuous nourishment, the heart muscle, like any other muscle, cannot function normally. When the blood flow to the heart becomes restricted because the coronary arteries are substantially, but not entirely, blocked, so that the heart muscle does not receive sufficient nourishment, it may become oxygen-deprived, a condition called *ischemia* (is-keem-iya), and warning signs called *angina* may occur (see below). If nourishment is diminished or cut off for a sufficient period of time, the muscle tissue or a portion of it may die. This is a heart attack.

A person suffering from ischemia is at some risk of a heart attack. The problem is, it is becoming clearer and clearer that not everyone experiences anginal pains when ischemia occurs. This condition is called *silent ischemia* and can best be detected when the person wears a monitoring device that continually tracks the electrocardial impulses and detects the conspicuous electrocardiogram (ECG) changes that occur when the heart muscle is starved for oxygen.

Angina Symptoms

The term angina describes the uncomfortable sensations that often occur when the heart is not receiving sufficient oxygen. Some individuals experience these sensations as pain, but others do not. Some of the symptoms include chest pains, breathlessness, pressure or heaviness beneath the sternum (breastbone); a feeling of tightness or constriction in the chest or arms; feelings of thickening or tightness in the throat; aches or feelings of numbness in the arms, throat, jaw, neck, shoulders, and back; and feelings of indigestion. These symptoms are warning signs that CAD exists. Often angina is experienced when the heart's demand for oxygen increases as, for example, during moments of physical activity or when the person is subjected to emotional stress. **Angina symptoms require medical attention.**

Factors Believed to Contribute to CAD

Heredity. Some individuals have been found to carry genes predisposing them to CAD; if you have a family history of heart attacks and heart disease among your parents and siblings, it is a possibility that you may be genetically predisposed to CAD and may need to institute lifestyle, dietary, and other changes to mitigate against such influences. In the future, it may be possible to identify individuals at high risk for CAD using molecular biological techniques because of the specific genes they may have inherited.

Gender. Although CAD is often considered to be a man's problem, it should be kept in mind that heart disease is the leading cause of death among women as well as men. Men appear to be more vulnerable to CAD than women, especially during the middle decades of life. Before the age of forty-five, men are about ten times more likely to have a heart attack than women are. Postmenopausal women appear to have an increased risk for CAD as compared to younger women. However, the risk for CAD among the former might be lowered by replacement estrogen treatment, which tends to raise the blood levels of the so-called "good" forms of cholesterol and lower the levels of the "bad" forms.

Smoking Cigarettes. This is a leading cause of cancer and heart disease, accounting for about 21 percent of all deaths from heart disease and among women about 41 percent of fatal heart attacks. A person who smokes more than doubles his or her risk for CAD. Persons who quit smoking appear to reduce their risk of CAD significantly.

High Blood Cholesterol Levels. Several major studies show a relationship between the level of cholesterol in the blood (spoken of as the serum cholesterol level) and the risk for CAD; the higher the levels, the greater the risk. Levels of total cholesterol above 200 milligrams per deciliter (mg/dl) have been found to increase CAD risk. A 1 percent reduction of serum cholesterol produces a 2 percent lowering in heart disease risk.

Diabetes. Diabetes is a disorder resulting from a disturbance of insulin production and, consequently, of sugar metabolism, which affects, among other things, the walls of the coronary arteries and increases the risk for damage to these arterial walls. This, in turn, increases the risk for CAD.

High Blood Pressure. High blood pressure, or hypertension, is considered to be present when the systolic blood pressure (the pressure in the arteries when the left ventricle contracts) is higher than 140 and the diastolic pressure (when the left ventricle relaxes) is higher than 90. Increased pressure seems to damage the artery walls and promotes CAD. Long-standing hypertension promotes the enlargement of the heart muscle cells, which, over time, may lead to a stiffening of the heart muscle and cause other problems, such as congestive heart failure and arrhythmias (abnormalities in the electrical impulses regulating the heart beat). Age, weight, chronic stress, for some people a high dietary salt intake, and other factors affect a person's blood pressure. Afro-Americans appear to have a higher risk for hypertension and its complications than Caucasians.

Body Weight. Overweight individuals have a higher risk for CAD than persons who are not overweight. The former also tend to have a higher incidence of diabetes, high blood pressure, and elevated blood cholesterol, all of which increase the risk for CAD even among individuals of appropriate body weight. Persons whose weight exceeds by 30 percent or more the desirable weight for their size and age are considered to be obese; being obese doubles one's risk of a heart attack.

Cholesterol is a fatty substance (lipid) that in small amounts is necessary to human life but which in excess tends to be deposited in the interior walls of the coronary arteries, contributing to the blockages involved in CAD. Because cholesterol is not water-soluble (hence not soluble in blood), it is circulated or transported attached to a protein molecule, forming a *lipoprotein* (lipid + protein). There are several types of lipoproteins, among which are: *low-density lipoproteins* (LDL), which tend to transport the cholesterol that deposits in the wall of the arteries; and *high-*

density lipoproteins (HDL), which take cholesterol from the body cells and transport it to the liver where it is broken down and eventually eliminated. Levels of LDL above 130 mg/dl of blood are associated with increased risks for CAD as are low levels of HDL. Levels of HDL (the so-called "good" form of cholesterol) of 36 mg/dl or higher are believed to *lower* the risk for CAD. According to recent guidelines, the LDL levels of persons with documented CAD, as for example anyone who has had a coronary bypass procedure, should be no higher than 100 mg/dl. Attached to lipoproteins are protein components known as *apolipoproteins*. Two such components, Apo B and Apo A-1, appear to be sensitive markers of CAD risk and may be used in the future to determine such risk. Another lipid-related substance is *Lp(a)*, a molecule composed of a glycoprotein (sugar + protein) attached to LDL. High levels of Lp(a) appear to be strongly associated with CAD. Current research suggests that LDL may be subdivided into classes of particles based on size. Smaller-sized particles of LDL seem to have a greater artery-blocking potential than larger-sized ones. Medically supervised megadoses of niacin may not only help lower Lp(a) levels but may be effective in elevating the proportion of relatively larger-sized LDL particles as well as HDL levels.

Sedentary Lifestyle. This is a major contributor to CAD since, by evolution, the human animal was meant to be active. Jane Brody, health editor of *The New York Times,* writes:

> Being physically active . . . could reduce risk of having a heart attack . . . by 35 to 55 percent from that of sedentary people of the same age. . . . Exercise enables the heart to work harder with less effort, . . . [lowers] the heart rate and blood pressure, increases the level

of . . . HDL, . . . decreases the tendency of the blood to form clots, minimizes the damage of stress on the heart and can help people lose excess weight.

Regular exercise also promotes an overall sense of psychological well-being. It's a winner!

Psychosocial Factors. These include chronic stress, anger and hostility, social isolation, and other psychological and behavioral issues that alone or in conjunction with any combination of the factors listed above are believed to promote CAD. Chronic stress and suppressed anger both seem to activate hormonal and physiological reactions that may affect the body's immune system and its ability to fight the buildup of fatty deposits in the arteries.

In an attempt to understand the psychological contribution to CAD, Drs. Meyer Friedman and Ray Rosenman in 1959 advanced the idea of the so-called *Type A personality.* According to these physicians, persons who were competitive, hard-driven, and high achievers, and who had a sense of time urgency or, as they put it, ". . . [were] aggressively involved in a chronic, incessant struggle to achieve more and more in less and less time . . . ," were especially prone to CAD. A *Type B personality* was also delineated and characterized as not exhibiting the Type A behaviors. Whatever merit these ideas had, they did unleash a large amount of research on psychological and behavioral variables in relation to heart disease. By the mid-1970s, two major longitudinal studies showed that Type A behaviors were associated with an increased incidence of CAD. However, when other studies could not confirm this association, attempts were made to elucidate what specific aspects of Type A behaviors may be more influential in the promotion of CAD. Many studies suggest that hostility and anger, particularly unexpressed anger, may be the essential factors in the risk of Type A behaviors.

ATHEROSCLEROSIS: HOW CAD DEVELOPS

For reasons entirely unknown even at this late date in human history, deposits of fat, cholesterol, and other substances begin to accumulate early in a person's life inside the arteries, at vulnerable points between the endothelial cells and the surrounding muscular tissue. This buildup, in vulnerable individuals, is believed to cause inflammatory reactions involving the white blood cells (which fight invading organisms or infections) and blood platelets, and results in swelling at the points of accumulation. As this process continues, plaques or lesions develop consisting of lipid material, scar tissue, and dead cells. Over time, calcium may be deposited into this material, making the plaque thicker and more rigid. Finally the plaque becomes sufficiently swollen to cause the inner endothelial layer to bulge and intrude into the arterial tube, thereby restricting blood flow. If this intrusion is sufficiently severe, total blockage or occlusion of the artery may occur. This entire process is referred to as atherosclerosis.

Atherosclerosis has often been referred to as hardening of the arteries, a term that reinforces the common misconception of the blood vessels as inert pipes through which the blood coursed. Instead, the blood vessels need to be thought of as a highly dynamic system that, due to hereditary and other factors, can malfunction because the body's normal defense mechanisms against infection and injury do not operate in the way they should at particular places in the circulatory system.

Recent research suggests that the inner lining of the arteries, the endothelial cells, plays a primary, if not the major, role in the process of atherosclerosis. Apparently the endothelial cells, which constitute an interface between the blood and the blood vessel walls, are involved in regulating blood pressure and blood-clotting processes. These cells produce a substance called an *endothelial-derived relaxing factor* (EDRF for short), which seems to counteract clot-promoting and vasoconstricting substances which are released by the blood platelets. Damage to, or the experimental removal of, the endothelial layer compromises the ability of the arterial walls to prevent or fight clot-formation and the progression of the atherosclerotic process.

Animal studies suggest that the edges of atherosclerotic plaques have an adhesion molecule that attracts and attaches to specialized white blood cells involved in the body's immune responses, called *macrophages.* Macrophages and other cells, called *T cells,* produce substances that kill foreign bacteria and help clean up debris at sites where inflammation or infection occurs. Macrophages also tend to oxidize low-density lipoprotein (LDL), the form of cholesterol associated with atherosclerosis. Apparently, oxidized LDL cholesterol is taken up by macrophages and, in addition, *attracts* macrophages to a growing atherosclerotic plaque. This results in the plaque's becoming clogged with cholesterol-laden macrophages, leading to further progression of the atherosclerotic process. In the future, the newly discovered adhesion molecule may come to serve as a marker for the early detection of atherosclerosis.

M E A S U R I N G   A R T E R I A L   B L O C K A G E

When blockage of the coronary arteries is suspected, as, for example, when the person is having symptoms of angina, a procedure known as *angiography* is frequently recommended.

Angiography enables doctors to "see" the condition of the coronary arteries. A thin, flexible catheter is painlessly inserted into an artery in an arm or leg and carefully guided under fluoroscopy into the aorta to the point at which the coronary arteries branch off. When the catheter is in position, a dye is injected through the catheter and a sequence of X-rays are taken. From these films an estimate of the degree of blockage or occlusion is generally made and the number and sites of blockage are determined.

The degree to which a coronary artery is blocked is generally communicated to patients in terms of percentages. "Your right coronary artery shows 75 percent occlusion whereas the left anterior descending coronary artery is 90 percent occluded." How does the cardiologist know this? Are precise measurements made? The answer to this last question is usually no. Except for research purposes, the numbers are the result of judicious eye-balling of the angiogram films. Certain arbitrary conventions are used. When the cardiologist looks at an angiogram, it is obvious when an artery is 100 percent blocked because no blood flow can be visualized where it normally should be seen. When the angiogram shows that the artery is constricted at some point by about three-fourths of its width, the cardiologist will probably tell you that it is 75 percent narrowed, or stenotic. If the artery is narrowed more than that but still shows some blood flow, it will probably be reported as 90 percent stenotic. If only a thin, narrow stream of blood flow is seen on the angiogram, the artery will probably be reported as being 99 percent blocked.

CAD may occur in one or all of the coronary arteries. When occlusions are found, most frequently the left anterior descending artery is involved. The right coronary artery and the circumflex arteries are involved less often and the left main, generally least of all. In general, multivessel involvement is more serious than when only one artery is involved. When all three major coronary arteries are involved, it is called *triple-vessel disease.*

TREATMENT OF CAD

When the coronary arteries are found to be blocked or partially blocked, one or more of several remedial procedures may be used. These include medications, angioplasty, and coronary bypass surgery.

Medications

Medications have not yet been developed that reverse the blockage of the coronary arteries. The more modest goal of medications is to improve the blood flow to and/or reduce the demand for oxygen in the heart muscle. Several different kinds of drugs are used to accomplish this.

Nitroglycerin. Perhaps the most common medication used for CAD is nitroglycerin, which comes in various forms, including tablets that can be dissolved under the tongue, liquids that can be injected intravenously or sprayed into the mouth, and patches that can be applied to the skin and that release a given amount of medicine slowly over a given period of time. Nitroglycerin is believed to work by reducing the size of the left ventricle and the muscle tension of the ventricle wall, decreasing its need for oxygen. This lowering of oxygen demand decreases the ischemia (oxygen starvation) and leads to the lessening of angina symptoms.

Beta-blockers. Beta-blockers are another group of medications used to treat CAD. The full name of these drugs is beta-adrenergic blocking agents, the adrenergic part referring to the adrenal hormones adrenalin (epinephrine) and noradrenalin (norepinephrine). These hormones are released by the adrenal glands when the organism perceives itself threatened or as being under stress. The major organs of the body, including the heart muscle and the walls of the blood vessels, have special receptor sites for these hormones. Thus, for example, when epinephrine is secreted when the organism perceives itself threatened, it attaches to receptor sites in the heart muscle and causes the heart to beat faster, thus preparing the organism for the "fight or flight" response. This means that the heart muscle requires more oxygen, just the condition that a person with angina symptoms does not want. Beta-blocking drugs are similar in chemical structure to the adrenal hormones and have the ability to lock on to adrenergic receptor sites; however, because of small differences in their chemical make-up, they do not have adrenergic capacities. When beta-blockers lock on to the receptor sites, the sites are not available for the real thing, the adrenal hormones. They are essentially blocked from responding in their usual way in the presence of the adrenergic hormones. Thus, beta-blockers slow down the heart rate, reducing the oxygen demand of the heart muscle.

Several studies suggest that the use of beta-blockers lowers the incidence of second heart attacks and sudden death by about 30 percent. Unfortunately, there are some undesirable side effects to beta-blockers. Some patients experience impotency and are unable to achieve or sustain an erection. Depression is another side effect.

Calcium Channel Blockers. A relatively new arrival on the medication scene is a group of drugs called calcium channel blockers. Calcium is necessary for muscle action. Contraction of muscle tissue is accomplished when calcium ions enter the muscle tissue by means of special channels in the membranes surrounding the muscle fiber. If these channels are blocked by drugs, muscle contraction can be reduced or eliminated. Calcium channel blockers slow or limit calcium entry into the smooth muscle of the coronary arteries, resulting in their dilatation or relaxation. They are particularly effective in the treatment of so-called angina at rest, which results from spasm of the coronary arteries.

Blood Thinners. Another medical approach is the use of so-called blood thinners. Actually, these drugs do not thin the blood or change its viscosity, they interfere with the chemical processes that lead to blood clotting (see below) and thus are really anticoagulants. A narrowed coronary artery appears to promote the growth of a thrombus (blood clot), which can block the artery, essentially cutting off blood flow and causing a heart attack. Some investigators believe that blood clotting may be involved in plaque formation in the coronary arteries. For unknown reasons, the plaque surface may become irregular or roughened and this may promote the formation of small blood clots that adhere to the plaque and, over time, increase the size of the plaque. In turn, this decreases the diameter of the artery. If the artery is sufficiently blocked, an additional clot may be enough to shut down all blood flow through the artery, causing a heart attack.

Blood-thinning agents, such as the drug Coumadin, act by interfering with the way the liver synthesizes the proteins involved in the clotting sequence. Other drugs, such as aspirin, act on the blood platelets, the cells that initiate and promote clot formation. When any tissue in the body sustains injury or tear, blood platelets stick to the injury and initiate the clotting reaction. This is a normal defense against bleeding after a tissue has sustained injury. The atherosclerotic plaques that build up in the coronary arteries may be vulnerable to microscopic bleeds. Platelets are believed to stick to the surface of the "bleeding" plaque, forming an ever-enlarging clump. Aspirin is believed to reduce the stickiness of blood platelets, thus reducing the chances that they will stick to irregular plaque surfaces and to each other. In turn, this reduces the chances of clot formation and subsequent plaque enlargement.

Recent research suggests that a baby aspirin a day may not only significantly decrease the chances of a second heart attack, but also reduce the chances of heart attack in persons with no history of CAD.

Balloon Angioplasty

A second major way of dealing with CAD is balloon angioplasty, a procedure developed in the mid-1970s. A catheter is inserted into the aorta to the opening of an obstructed coronary artery, as in routine angiography. Then a guide wire is passed through the catheter to the site of the obstruction in the artery. When the guide wire is positioned properly, a catheter with a balloon at its tip is passed along the guide wire. The balloon is inflated and, under pressure, the plaque is squashed flat against the artery wall, leaving, it is hoped, an adequate channel for blood flow.

Not every person with CAD is automatically a candidate for angioplasty. This procedure appears to work best when one or two coronary arteries are involved. If all three major coronary arteries are substantially blocked, it would be riskier to attempt the procedure, which requires shutting off blood flow temporarily in an artery in order to inflate the balloon. The location and size of the plaques may also play a role in determining whether or not the angioplasty procedure can be used.

The chance of successfully dilating an artery at a point where it is occluded is about 90 percent, and the risk for a major complication occurring is about 4 percent. Heart attack and death related to the procedure is low. However, sometimes during the procedure an artery occludes completely and this may require placement of a stent (see p. 37) or being rushed to the operating room for bypass surgery in order to prevent a heart attack.

Another point for consideration is that there is about a 30 to 40 percent chance that the coronary artery "opened up" via angioplasty will close down again within twelve months (restenosis). Despite these problems, the fact that surgery might be avoided has made the angioplasty procedure a preferred treatment in many cases of CAD. In 1983, about 30,000 angioplasty procedures were performed in the United States. In 1990, it is estimated that more than 266,000 procedures were done.

Bypass Surgery

The third major remedial approach to CAD is bypass surgery, which involves removing parts of other blood vessels and using them to create a detour—or bypass—around the blocked portions of coronary arteries. The most commonly used blood vessel "grafts" are the saphenous vein in the leg and the internal mammary arteries that come off the aorta and feed the shoulder and chest areas. The graft vein is sewn on one end to an opening made in the aorta and on the other end to one of the coronary arteries (see Figure 4, page 31). Because the internal mammary artery is already attached to the aorta, only its distal or far end needs to grafted to the coronary artery, downstream from the blocked portion.

According to the latest statistics, the number of individuals receiving bypass surgery increases each year. In 1991, more than 400,000 such operations were done in the United States. Overall, three to four times more men have the operation than women. In one study in Atlanta, Georgia, about half of the persons electing to have bypass surgery had not had a previous heart attack, and of those who had had a heart attack, about 72.3 percent also elected to have bypass surgery. Only about 13.7

CORONARY ARTERY DISEASE **Figure 4**

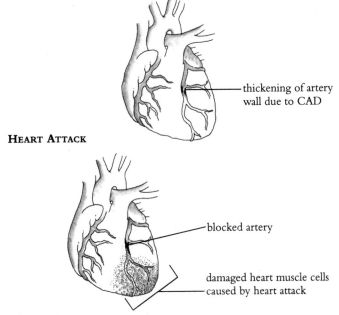

thickening of artery
wall due to CAD

HEART ATTACK

blocked artery

damaged heart muscle cells
caused by heart attack

When blood flow to the myocardium is suddenly blocked by a blood clot, a heart attack occurs. This can cause part of the heart muscle supplied by the artery to die.

ARTERY GRAFT

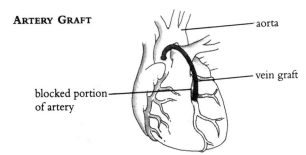

aorta

vein graft

blocked portion
of artery

To restore blood flow to the heart, a surgeon uses a vein from the thigh or calf or an artery from the chest wall as a graft. One end of the graft is attached beyond the obstruction, and the other is attached to the aorta. This creates a new route for the flow of blood.

percent of all the patients needed bypass surgery on an emergency basis.

Bypass surgery was developed in the early 1960s. Because it is so relatively new as a treatment for CAD, hearsay and misunderstanding abounds about its safety, efficacy, and associated rate of medical complications (morbidity) and mortality. Several studies have attempted to demonstrate that persons who have bypass surgery have fewer symptoms of angina and survive longer than individuals treated only with medications. Perhaps the most famous study, conducted several decades ago, is a collaborative effort called the Coronary Artery Surgery Study (CASS). This study found that bypass surgery was effective in reducing anginal symptoms. About 25 percent of patients with triple vessel disease (the term used when all three main coronary arteries are affected) were free of angina when treated with medications alone, whereas 70 to 80 percent of those who had the bypass procedure were symptom-free. However, the CASS researchers did not find that bypass surgery had any advantage over medications in increasing survival rates. They found the two approaches to be equivalent; about 90 percent of those in each group were alive five years after the beginning of their respective treatments.

Since the CASS research was carried out, there have been major improvements in operating room techniques and postoperative aftercare and the baseline rates of complications (morbidity) and mortality associated with bypass surgery have been substantially reduced. Several researchers now believe that the CASS data are irrelevant to the current situation and that patients undergoing bypass surgery are living longer as compared to patients in earlier years. In one recent study, carried out at Duke University Medical Center, followup of patients revealed that "patients undergoing [bypass] surgery in the 1980s are living significantly longer than surgical patients in the previous decade."

A followup of patients revealed that at each time point between two and ten years, patients who had bypass surgery survived at higher rates than patients treated only with medications. Who is a candidate for coronary bypass surgery? Any individual with left main coronary artery involvement, that is, with significant blockage of the left coronary artery before it divides into two; blockage there would affect a major portion of the heart muscle. Other prime candidates are persons with severe triple vessel disease and/or individuals who do not seem to improve with angioplasty or medication. In the Duke University study, followup after seven years showed that of the patients with left main disease, over 80 percent of those who had bypass surgery had survived whereas only about 38 percent of the medically treated group were still alive.

Risks Associated with Bypass Surgery. What are the risks of bypass surgery? The major immediate risk is not surviving the surgery. The overall risk of surgical mortality was about 1.6 percent in the CASS study. Persons over sixty-five years of age had a surgical mortality risk about three times higher (4.8 percent), generally because of the increasing likelihood of other medical problems, such as diabetes, other circulatory problems, etc. Individuals who have already had a heart attack have an obviously higher surgical mortality rate than those who have not had a heart attack. Women, for unknown reasons, seem to have greater difficulty with bypass surgery than men do. Compared to men, they tend to have a higher surgical mortality rate, the patency of the grafts is not as successful, and postoperative relief from anginal symptoms seems to be less. Moreover, women seem to recover more slowly and have relatively more difficulties in psychosocial adjustments after bypass surgery than men do. It was thought that the fact that women as a group tend to be older than men when they have heart attacks and/or their coronary arteries were smaller than those of men might explain these gender differences. But a more recent study in which age differences were taken into account still showed higher death rates and poorer prognosis after bypass surgery among women.

Some of the other risks of bypass surgery that need to be considered are the possibility of a heart attack's occurring during surgery and the possibility of loosening a blood clot that then travels to the brain and causes a stroke. These latter risks, fortunately, are low. A more problematic issue is the possibility that the new grafts do not remain open, or patent—that is, for unknown reasons they close up prematurely. The CASS research found that over half of the vein grafts used in bypass surgery tended to clog up in about ten years or so. This led to the greater utilization of the internal mammary artery (IMA) as graft material because it tends to hold up longer than the venous grafts. On average, between 85 and 90 percent of the IMA grafts remained open after ten years. This translates into improved survival, fewer angina episodes, and fewer reoperations.

It needs to be kept in mind that most studies have not controlled for such variables as changes in lifestyle (reduced fat/cholesterol intake, reduced stress, and/or increased exercise) and the impact of such changes on the duration of vein or artery grafts. Recent evidence suggests that men who had bypass surgery and were treated with cholesterol-lowering drugs and a diet low in fat and cholesterol showed fewer adverse changes in their bypass grafts and fewer new blockages than men treated with placebos and less rigorous dietary restrictions. The question remains whether or not, after bypass surgery, changes in lifestyle without medication can achieve results comparable to medication treatment.

The Bypass Procedure. Bypass surgery requires the services of a team of specialists. Once the hair of the chest, abdomen, pubic area, and legs has been shaved, the first specialist, the anesthesiologist, takes charge. Although specific procedures may vary somewhat from center to center, in general the anesthesiologist inserts various intravenous lines into the patient's hands and/or arm(s) through which anesthetic agents and other fluids are administered or blood pressure monitored during the surgery. Also, once the patient is anesthetized, he or she will insert a tube past the larynx, where the vocal cords are located, into the trachea (windpipe). This endotracheal tube is connected to a breathing machine and regulates the breathing throughout the procedure. Several other catheters are also inserted into the veins of the neck. These provide moment-to-moment information about blood pressure and can be used to administer various drugs directly to the heart. A catheter is also inserted into the urethra through which the urine is drained.

Once all the tubes and monitoring leads are in place, the surgeons take over. Attention is given to two areas of the body: a leg or legs and the chest. Following an incision into the leg, a section of the saphenous vein is removed and the ends remaining are sutured. This vein is a relatively strong one and is generally capable of withstanding the pressures required of the arterial blood vessels. Meanwhile, work on the chest has begun. A lengthwise incision is made down the breastbone, which is literally cut in half and pulled apart. When the surgery is complete, the sternum will be wired back together and, for all intents and purposes, will be as strong as new. If the left mammary artery is going to be utilized in the bypass procedure, this is exposed at this time.

The next phase of the procedure is to connect the patient to a heart-lung machine, truly one of the most awe-inspiring pieces of medical technology ever created. In order to operate on the coronary arteries, it is necessary to still the beating of the heart. This can be accomplished with drugs once the major blood vessels are hooked up to the heart-lung machine, which, as its name implies, takes over the functions of both the heart and the lungs. The heart-lung machine keeps the blood circulating through the body while the surgery proceeds. In addition, the circulating blood itself is cooled down to about 25 degrees Celsius (77 degrees Fahrenheit). When the body tissue is cooled, its oxygen requirements are diminished. This cooling also contributes to the postsurgical pallor of the patient.

The longer the patient remains on the heart-lung machine, the greater the opportunity for something going amiss during the course of the surgery. Thus, the surgical team is ever mindful of the time elapsing in the course of the surgery and, sometimes, the benefits of making specific vessel grafts have to be weighed against the risks accruing because of the amount of time spent on the heart-lung machine.

The surgeon in charge of the bypass also needs to make other decisions. For example, the number of bypasses or grafts that are made is often decided on during the surgery. The angiogram gives the surgeon only a rough idea of where the blocks are, how severe they might be, the diameter of the arteries available for a grafting procedure, and so on. The actual situation has to be reassessed when the patient is "opened up." The operation will be referred to as a triple, quadruple, or even quintuple bypass, depending on the number of bypasses that are made.

If the bypass graft is from the saphenous vein, it is sewn on one end to the aorta and on the other end to a place on one of the coronary arteries so that the occluded portion of the artery is literally bypassed. In other words, the blood flow from the aorta now has an alternative pathway to bring blood to the heart muscle. Over time, the occluded artery tends to seal off completely so that blood flow occurs only through the new graft. In a similar fashion, if the internal mammary artery is being used, it is severed at its normal attachment to the shoulder area and grafted to one of the coronary arteries (its other end is already attached to the aorta). When the bypass grafts are all in place and tested out, the patient is weaned off the heart-lung machine and the heart beat is restarted. When the heart action is sufficiently stable, the patient is completely removed from the heart-lung machine and the process of closing up begins.

The closing-up process requires the installation of several tubes to drain the heart area and the chest. Once the tubes are in place, the sternum is wired together and the final suturing is done. The incision in the leg from which the vein was removed is stapled together and then wrapped in elastic gauze. When this process is finished the patient is placed on a gurney and taken to the recovery room, where he/she is hooked up to multiple monitoring devices. From beginning to end the surgery may last three or more hours.

Other Techniques for Treating CAD

In recent years, several new techniques have been developed for dealing with CAD, but relative to angioplasty or bypass surgery they are not yet widely available. Attempts have been made to implant delicate wire mesh tubes into blocked coronary arteries to hold the clogging deposits of plaque against the artery wall. These tubes, called *coronary artery stents,* have been used in more than a thousand patients in the United States over the past few years, but their effectiveness is still unproven. A *New England Journal of Medicine* article reported that six months after implantation nearly half of the arteries that were opened had closed down again. However, more recent studies are more promising and the use of stents is becoming an increasingly successful option, especially as a "bridge" between angioplasty and bypass surgery. Other techniques being tested include the use of lasers and of cutters that burn, shave, or drill their way through the plaque in clogged arteries. The safety and effectiveness of these procedures need to be documented. One promising procedure is *artherectomy*, which has recently been approved by the FDA for treatment of CAD. Originally developed to remove the plaque buildup in the arteries of the legs, it was applied to the coronary arteries in 1987. Since then, about 145,000 persons have been treated worldwide. The procedure is similar to balloon angioplasty except that whereas in balloon angioplasty the plaque is compressed to the arterial wall, in artherectomy the plaque is literally drilled through and removed. The risk for restenosis of the arteries appears to be about the same as for angioplasty. However, the impression is that the risk of emergency bypass as a complication of the procedure may be lower than that for angioplasty.

SUGGESTED READING

Altman, L. K. 1991. Unraveling the mystery of bypass survival. *The New York Times,* August 20, p. B6.

American Heart Association. 1981. Coronary artery bypass graft surgery. Publ. No. 50-047A.

American Heart Association. 1993. Heart and stroke facts. Publ. No. 55-0514 (com).

Brody, J. E. 1992. Understanding, and controlling, risks can help lower chance of heart attack. *The New York Times,* July 22, p. B7.

Halperin, J. L., and R. Levine. 1985. *Bypass.* New York: Random House.

Horovitz, E. 1988. *Heart Beat.* Los Angeles: Health Trend Publ.

Marx, J. 1990. Holding the line against heart disease. *Science* 248: 1491–1493.

Motulsky, A. G. 1991. Lipid risk factors in coronary heart disease: Emergence of Lp(a). *Genome* 2: 1–2.

Pearson, T., E. Rapaport, M. Criqui, et al. 1994. Optimal risk factor management in the patient after coronary revascularization: A statement for healthcare professionals from an American Heart Association Writing Group. *Circulation* 90: 3125–3133.

Pryor, D. B., F. E. Harrell, Jr., J. S. Rankin, et al. 1987. The changing survival benefits of coronary revascularization over time. *Circulation* 76 (suppl V): V13–V21.

Superko, H. R. 1989. Drug therapy and the prevention of atherosclerosis in humans. *Am. Jour. of Cardiology* 64: 31G–38G.

Yalof, I. 1983. *Open Heart Surgery.* New York: Random House.

Two

. . . .

PREPARING FOR SURGERY:
PRACTICAL AND PHYSICAL
CONSIDERATIONS

T his chapter is addressed largely to the person who chooses bypass surgery on an elective basis. Here, the patient often has a broad range of options as to where the surgery will be done, which surgeon will perform it and so on, and the luxury of time in which to make the necessary decisions. If time is short or if you are a friend or relative of an individual undergoing emergency bypass surgery, turn to the end of the chapter (page 57) for some basic pointers that might be of help to you.

GET A SECOND OPINION

If possible, before you decide to have bypass surgery obtain a second opinion about its necessity. Medical records and angiogram films are available to the patient and may be brought or sent by some sort of overnight delivery service to other physicians for review. If one physician advises surgery and a second one advises against it, or if you still remain ambivalent about surgery, do not hesitate to seek a third opinion. Many second-opinion insurance programs will pay for a third opinion under such conditions.

DO YOUR HOMEWORK

Once the decision to proceed with bypass surgery has been made, consider (or reconsider) your choices regarding the surgeon and the hospital. Since your life is at stake, these decisions need to be made carefully. It is amazing how often such choices are made on the basis of hearsay or arbitrary information rather than on rational, well-thought-out personal research. The same person who might spend hours agonizing over a decision about which tie or dress to buy might spend fewer than ten seconds thinking about a decision on which his or her life might depend. One person I spoke to chose his surgeon on the basis of the fact that a friend of his had survived surgery performed by the surgeon several years earlier. He said, "He saved my friend's life. I wouldn't use anyone else." No thought was given to the possibility that the surgeon might not be performing bypass surgery as frequently anymore (and might be rusty), that he or she might now be impaired in some way, or that his or her reputation might have declined since the friend was operated on.

You need to remember that the surgeon has other chances to learn from his/her mistakes whereas you have only one life to live. So careful, thoughtful, and deliberate choice should be a major priority.

When it comes to major surgery, everyone wants the best surgeon to do it at the finest hospital. Some individuals actually have the financial and other resources to travel anywhere to get the most up-to-date and superior medical treatment money can buy. Most of us, however, are limited in this regard and have to make do with what's available in our particular locality and/or our particular medical group, health maintenance organization, and insurance plan. But even with such limitations, there are probably more choices available to us than we realize, and that makes it necessary to do some homework before proceeding with the surgery.

CHOOSING A LOCALE

In thinking about a locale or a specific hospital, consider whether or not it is important to you to be close to your social support system—family and friends. This system of support frequently plays a major role in maintaining morale and aiding the healing process. If you elect to have surgery in a locale where friends and relatives can't be present on a regular basis, you may be cutting yourself off from needed psychological support, particularly in the immediate postsurgical period. Research on the effects of social support and recovery from bypass surgery strongly suggests that patients who receive such support while in the hospital tend to require less pain medication and to recover faster (as measured by a shorter stay in intensive care and overall in the hospital) after surgery than patients with meager support.

There may be good reasons to choose a more distant locale in which to have surgery rather than a closer one. For example, your local hospital may have an unacceptably high rate of postsurgical problems (such information is generally available from your local Department of Health). Also, by choosing a close-by locale, you may be limiting your choice of surgeons and/or hospitals.

CHOOSING A SURGEON

Once the decision about general locale is made, it is time to choose a surgeon. Surgeons must be affiliated with a hospital in order to perform surgery there, and many surgeons are affiliated with only one or two hospitals; thus, by choosing the surgeon one often narrows down the choice of hospital.

At least once or twice a year, an article appears in the newspaper or in the popular magazines on the subject of how to choose a competent doctor or surgeon. Almost invariably, these articles emphasize the same few points. For example, they all say to choose someone who is board-certified in their area of specialty. Generally, but not always, competence and board certification go hand in hand. Unfortunately, it isn't so easy to ascertain the information that would demonstrate competence. A recent study concluded that it was virtually impossible even for professionals to obtain access to complete and verifiable information about a physician and his/her competency. In response to public demand, the American Board of Medical Specialties set up a hotline (1-800-776-2378) to provide information on the board certification status of a physician. Once you have a list of possible surgeons, you might also want to check their listings in a book called the *ABMS Compendium of Certified Medical Specialists,* available in the reference department of most major libraries.

A layperson is at a disadvantage in assessing the competence of a given doctor or medical facility. Even professionals have difficulty in assessing other professionals, particularly outside their own domain of expertise. For example, as a psychotherapist, I "know" about the reputation and competency of some of my fellow therapists in the area where I live and practice. Some of the information comes from firsthand experience of having worked with, observed, or otherwise interacted and personally assessed the other person. Some of my information comes secondhand from what other therapists and/or clients have told me. Thus, assessing the competency of a colleague is hardly a scientific endeavor. It's a question of judgment arrived at by sifting through and weighing personal experiences and the opinions and biases of others.

Probably the best way to find a "good" surgeon—i.e., one with an excellent reputation and considered by others as qualified and competent—is to ask other physicians. It may not be the best way to judge competence but, given that there probably isn't any "best" way, it may be the only way open to most people. A good starting point is to ask your primary-care physician for a list of competent surgeons. If he/she cannot come up with an immediate list, put your doctor to work for you. Ask him/her to check around with colleagues and come up with some recommendations. A doctor who cares about your health and welfare should be willing to do that much for you.

Another starting point is your insurance company. They may have lists of surgeons (as well as hospitals) that they approve of in your area. Insurance companies sometimes have preferred providers lists and to become a preferred provider a physician has had to submit documentation of board certification, etc. Thus, some of the legwork has already been done for you. Of course, do not expect your insurance company to recommend any one surgeon or medical facility. That would not be ethical. They may, however, tell you which surgeons may require you to obtain a second opinion and which would not, and that should count for something. Be aware, too, that your insurance company may have more of a vested interest in referring you to the surgeon with the lowest fees than the one who will necessarily do the best job.

Other suggestions include the following:

• Call up your local medical association or medical center and ask for their advice.

• Call up several cardiologists and ask them, "If you or a member of your family needed bypass surgery, whom would you go to to have it done?" (Suggest this question to your doctor if he or she is going to do the inquiries for you.) See which names come up most frequently.

* If you need the names of cardiologists to call, look in the Yellow Pages under the heading of Physicians and the subheading, Cardiology. (Do not, by the way, choose a surgeon or a personal physician solely on the basis of his or her Yellow Pages listing. Always check out their credentials and competence through other sources.)

When you call a physician, expect that the receptionist or nurse will try to "protect" the "boss" and might intervene so that you never get to speak to the person you are calling. Simply insist that you must talk to the doctor. Leave your phone number, if necessary, so that he or she can call you back. Tell the receptionist or nurse you need the doctor's advice, and emphasize the word *doctor*.

If you have physician friends, do not hesitate to ask their advice. Physicians in general have access to a broader range of doctors, cardiologists, and surgeons than most laypersons would ever be able to amass. Most important, they have access to information about the reputations and "classified" scuttlebutt about particular cardiovascular surgeons that medical associations and insurance companies could not, and would not pass on to a layperson.

Interview the Candidates. I strongly suggest that, once you have a list of names, you personally interview each surgeon on the list. Start with a list of no more than three names, otherwise the task of interviewing becomes overwhelming. If none of the three seems right, make up another list of two or three names. Let the candidates know that you are engaged in the process of finding a surgeon and intend to interview several.

Make up a list in advance of questions that you need answered. Some examples are: Where were you trained? How many years have you been in practice? How many bypass procedures do you perform each year? In which hospitals do you perform surgery? A more exhaustive list of questions appears at the end of the chapter (page 55).

You want a surgeon with lots of current experience in performing coronary bypass operations. Such doctors tend to have the best track records in terms of operative mortality and complications. You also want someone you can talk to, someone who deals with you and your spouse with respect and dignity. And, of course, you want someone who inspires confidence and trust.

As you talk to the surgeon, *be aware of how he or she treats you.* Does he or she respect your need to shop around? You have every right to do so, and if the surgeon does not approve of your shopping strategy, it may spell communication difficulties between the two of you further down the line. You want someone who is professionally secure and is not threatened by your questions and your need to shop for a surgeon.

Also *note whether or not he or she employs scare techniques to drive you to the operating table.* One surgeon I interviewed casually mentioned that my left coronary artery was 99 percent occluded, whereas every other doctor to whom I spoke put the figure at no higher than 90 percent. It is a small matter and of no great significance in real terms. However, it left an aftertaste in my mouth and a distinct impression that he was trying to frighten me into a decision I was not yet ready to make. From my discussions with other persons who have had bypass surgery, it seems that many were subjected to scare tactics by their cardiologists and surgeons. Many physicians are simply unaware that they are employing such tactics and, if asked, would deny that they are doing so. Some physicians, however, will admit that, when asked by patients when the surgery should be done, they tend to recommend a delay of no more than a few days. In short, the timing is often presented in a way that leaves the patient believing that time is of the essence and that the problem is so severe and urgent that it cannot be put off. I suspect that many physicians just do not understand what impact such statements of urgency can have on a person already concerned or frightened over the diagnosis of atherosclerosis. It tends to rob the patient of a sense of choice.

One physician I spoke to admitted that he tends to "push" the scheduling of the surgery because he believes that the longer the decision is put off, the harder it becomes for the patient to commit to the procedure. Also, physicians tend to be overly concerned about liability issues and do not want to be accused later on by the patient (or his/her survivors) of not "warning" them of the possibility of a heart attack's occurring before the surgery is scheduled.

In interviewing surgeons, also *assess whether or not a particular candidate respects your knowledge and the fact that you might have done some homework before coming to see him or her.* In other words, does he or she listen to you? One surgeon I interviewed used simplistic terms in describing the bypass procedure. Whenever I asked questions, I tended to use the technical terms (e.g., the anatomical names of the specific blood vessels) since I had extensive education in this field and at one time taught courses in comparative anatomy. It wasn't a question of showing off my knowledge; it was just the way I thought about the matter. The surgeon showed no awareness of my knowledge and continued to use simplistic rather than more sophisticated terms. Again, this is a small matter. But it told me that this doctor does not listen well to his patients and that this might pose a problem in our relationship later on.

Although a surgeon with integrity would not perform unnecessary surgery, do not expect a surgeon to give you an objective assessment as to whether or not you need surgery. Nevertheless, *if you have doubts about surgery, raise the question with the surgeon you are interviewing and see how he or she handles the question.* Does he or she respect your ambivalence or doubts? Does he or she move into a sales mode and try to sell you on the idea of surgery rather than providing understanding and empathy? Does he or she help you resolve your ambivalence and/or reach a decision while respecting your autonomy?

Also assess how the surgeon treats your spouse or significant other. This is not a small matter. Almost all the spouses of bypass patients I talked with had some complaint about the way cardiologists and surgeons treated or related to them, especially if the spouse was a woman and the surgeon a man. Women tended to report that when they interviewed a male surgeon together with their patient mates, their questions tended to go unanswered and their presence was ignored. In such circumstances, spouses tend to feel snubbed and are left with few positive feelings toward the surgeon. The surgeon I finally chose recognized that my wife and I tended to work together as a unit, and thus he treated Hilda with equal consideration and respect. For example, he reviewed the angiogram films in our presence, recognizing that it was highly likely that she had never seen these films. He treated her questions with the same sobriety and seriousness as those I raised. Thus, in his behavior and demeanor he communicated to us that he would be able to deal effectively with both of us.

Assess what kind of mood you are in after talking to the surgeon. Did he or she depress you, or were you left feeling uplifted? One of the surgeons I interviewed seemed to have a depressive style and, given my own mental state during the period just after I received the diagnosis of CAD, I needed someone more upbeat and positive. In any case, this particular physician was patronizing and never acknowledged the knowledge I had obtained from my reading and from my discussions with other physicians. He was quickly eliminated from consideration. Another surgeon seemed to be a nice fellow, knowledgeable and competent, but the chemistry was not right. There was no inner voice screaming, "That's the one." When I asked around among some physician friends about his reputation I was informed that over the past few years he had specialized in heart valve transplant surgery and was not doing as many bypass procedures. That eliminated him. I wanted someone who could do a bypass procedure in his sleep.

CHOOSING A HOSPITAL

If choosing a surgeon is a heroic task, what should be said about choosing the hospital where the surgery will be performed. On what basis should the choice be made? One might call a series of hospitals and ascertain the mortality (death) rate and the rate of postsurgical complications (morbidity). In my particular locale, the average mortality rate was between 1 and 2 percent (state departments of health generally maintain such statistics); however, in some communities the rates of morbidity and mortality might vary considerably between hospitals.

Some surgical teams operate at several hospitals. I found that at one local hospital with an excellent reputation the team had a rate considerably higher than the average; while at a second hospital the same team had an average rate of postsurgical mortality and complications. On inquiry I discovered that the more difficult, high-risk cases were generally operated on in the first hospital whereas the more routine cases were handled at the second one.

The quality of the postsurgical team, nursing and otherwise, may also contribute to the rate of mortality and morbidity, and it would be wise to inquire about the pre- and postsurgical support staff. One of the factors apparently contributing to survival following bypass surgery is the quality of nursing care. Inquire about the ratio of nurses to patients in the immediate postsurgical period. Optimally, this should be one to one, because if a complication occurs following surgery, the nurse is likely to be the one to initiate remedial measures. This may result in saving the patient's life.

Discuss these issues with the surgeon you select and consider the advice he or she gives carefully, particularly if he or she has worked with several surgical and postsurgical teams at different medical centers. If there are major discrepancies in morbidity/mortality rates at the hospitals in your locality, also discuss this matter with your surgeon before committing yourself to having the surgery in a specific hospital.

Another choice that might be open to you is that of a teaching hospital, as opposed to a private, nonteaching hospital. There are distinct differences of opinion about the benefits of each. Some individuals seem to require the prestige of a big-name medical center to feel safe and secure for their particular surgery. And for some kinds of surgery, such major medical centers are the only place to go because it is there one can find the experienced physicians for that type of surgery. But teaching hospitals do not necessarily have the best surgical and postsurgical setup or personnel. For bypass surgery, which is now a fairly routine operation, you might receive more personalized and attentive care at a local community hospital.

If you decide to have your surgery at a teaching hospital, find out who, specifically, will be holding the scalpel and doing the procedure. Will your surgeon be supervising a resident in training, or will he or she be the actual hands-on surgeon? In my particular case, I had a choice between two institutions: a teaching hospital and a private nonteaching hospital. The same surgery at the first hospital would, according to the surgeon, take almost a full hour longer than at the second one due to the teaching needs of observing students. Keeping in mind that a longer surgery requires more anesthesia and increases the risks to the patient, I chose the nonteaching hospital. In addition, I knew from other physicians that there were many personnel problems and turnover at the teaching facility. I had no problem in this particular choice.

Make inquiries about the morale of the personnel at a given hospital. In one situation, during an interview of a surgeon at a local hospital, he suggested that I wait a week before being admitted because the X-ray technicians were on strike and would, it was hoped, be back to work the next week. The strike might end, but the feelings engendered by such actions might not, and might interfere with high-quality care later on.

OTHER TASKS TO ACCOMPLISH BEFORE SURGERY

Once you've decided on a surgeon and hospital, and have set the date for admission, it's time to ensure that other important details are in place.

First, decide (with your significant other) who has to know about your surgery. Do not be surprised if your anxiety level increases after you tell your friends, employer, and family members about the forthcoming surgery. The news may arouse other people's anxieties and fears, which, in turn, may "infect" you. In some instances, as the news of a person's surgery makes the rounds of his or her social circle, the person's telephone may not stop ringing as each member of the circle calls to find out what happened and possibly to extend best wishes. (An answering machine may help to control the flood of calls in this situation.) This, in itself, may increase your anxiety or that of your significant other if you are unprepared for it. Also, your "problem" may trigger memories of other people's experiences, some of which may be irrelevant to your situation or your needs. Remind yourself that people generally want to help, and want you to know that they care about what happens to you.

In some subcultures, it would not be polite to limit or place constraints on other people's show of respect and caring when they call. Thus, in spite of the anxiety such conversations might arouse, the patient is expected and "required" to play a special role in accepting the well wishes of others. Each person or couple needs to make a decision about the degree to which they can tolerate their own and others' anxieties, and plan accordingly.

Second, be sure you have executed your medical power of attorney forms, and that your surgeon and primary physician both have copies of the document. Should something go wrong during or following surgery, you may not want to have your life prolonged or the doctors to attempt medical heroics if the quality of your life is going to be hopelessly compromised. In my case, I made my exact wishes known to my wife and children so that my family and physicians could act on my behalf when I could no longer do so. These are generally not easy issues to deal with, but once the unpleasant possibilities are out in the open and talked about, and once everyone's feelings are expressed, the issue is over with, taken care of. The mind becomes free to deal with other important matters.

Third, be sure your will is in good order. Attorneys are often able to cooperate when time is short and documents need to be prepared or altered quickly. Fax machines and overnight delivery services have made life simpler in this regard. Remind yourself that the more completely you take care of the business end of life and death, the more energy you will have available for such matters as preparing for the surgery itself.

Fourth, the period before surgery is an appropriate time to make your wishes known to family and friends as to burial, cremation, and so on. Some individuals seem to think it is depressing, morbid, or fatalistic to think about such matters just before major surgery. Giving voice to these issues might be taken to mean you have given up on life and expect not to survive the surgery. I do not share these views. Verbalizing is the way to defuse emotionally charged thoughts, to make them manageable and less frightening and powerful. Thus, discussing the possibility of death and one's wishes about the arrangements afterward is a way of experiencing greater control over an unpleasant, perhaps frightening, prospect, and of mastering one's feelings. It also tends to give you the sense that you are a responsible adult. It means you are coping with reality. One thing is certain: *Not* thinking about the possibility of dying during or immediately after surgery in no way guarantees your survival. Evidence in health psychology suggests that facing rather than avoiding one's fears tends to help mobilize inner and external resources so that survival is promoted.

Fifth, arrange for blood donors in case you need a transfusion during or after the surgery. Of course, you could just take whatever blood was available, if it came to that. Screening for hepatitis and AIDS has made blood transfusions much safer today than they were just a short time ago. However, if you want an additional margin of safety and if you have the time, you can donate designated units of your own blood in advance of surgery. This is the absolute best blood to use if you need a transfusion. However, surgeons are reluctant to have you give blood just before you have surgery. You need all that blood because you will surely lose some of it during the surgery. If you have months to spare prior to surgery, then you have the time to have units of blood set aside. However, one does not always have that much leeway.

The second-best solution is to have friends and relatives of your ABO and rhesus blood type designate blood for you. This requires time and energy to recruit donors who may have to go some distance to the appropriate blood bank to give blood in your name. But friends are frequently eager to help out in this matter. Among other reasons, it makes them feel less helpless in the face of an upsetting event over which they have no control. Also, they feel part of the process of healing you. Many of my friends were disappointed that they could not donate blood because they did not have the right ABO blood type. Some of them had organized a carpool to go to the blood bank, only to discover that the majority of them were not of the blood type I needed. It was the thought that counted.

THINGS TO DO TO PREPARE FOR SURGERY

1. Obtain a second opinion about the necessity of surgery if you have the time to do so.

2. Obtain the names of surgeons from your physician(s) and make a list of those you want to interview.

3. Schedule interviews (see sample questions below) and choose a surgeon who inspires confidence and with whom you can talk comfortably.

4. Decide on a date for the surgery with your surgeon.

5. Choose the hospital where the surgery will be done.

6. Inform relatives and friends about your decision.

7. Check to see that your will and power of attorney for health matters—indicating your wishes regarding life-prolonging measures—are in order and, if not, put them right.

8. Discuss your wishes with your spouse and/or family regarding the possibility of not surviving the surgery; talking about dying does not cause death, and facing and overcoming one's fears may promote your survival.

9. Arrange to have blood designated for your use during surgery if you have the time to do so; this is often done in conjunction with the hospital at which the surgery occurs.

10. Arrange a telephone tree in advance so that the task of informing friends and relatives about the outcome of the surgery can be shared.

QUESTIONS TO ASK A PROSPECTIVE SURGEON

1. Where were you trained and are you board-certified?

2. How many years have you been in practice?

3. How many bypass procedures did you perform in the past year?

4. What are your personal rates of success in bypass surgery in terms of survival and complications?

5. How do you account for the difference in your success rate and those of other surgeons?

6. Who else is part of your surgical team?

7. Who will actually be operating on me?

8. In your opinion, is this surgery really necessary? Are there alternatives I might consider?

9. What benefits might I expect from the surgery?

10. How much aftercare will you provide?

11. In which hospitals do you perform surgery?

12. Which hospital would you recommend, and why?

13. Which hospital in your opinion has the best postsurgical team?

14. What are the usual complications in the postsurgical period?

15. How often will I see you in the hospital after the surgery?

16. How long do you expect I'll be hospitalized?

17. What are the most common complications I might expect?

18. What are your fees?

19. Have you ever had surgery yourself?

20. How do you keep up-to-date on the latest techniques and advances?

21. Are there any other surgeons you recommend I speak to?

IN CASE OF EMERGENCY BYPASS SURGERY

Emergency bypass surgery usually results from either difficulties encountered in the course of balloon angioplasty or from a heart attack. In the former instance, the prudent patient may have prepared for the possibility of bypass surgery before going into angioplasty; if a bypass becomes necessary it will be done on the spot.

When the patient has had a heart attack and is informed that surgery is immediately necessary, there will probably be only a very little time for preparation and choices will be limited. In this instance, it is helpful if someone is available to be an advocate—if possible, the patient's spouse or significant other, or a friend; otherwise, a nurse—to help in the decision-making. For example, the advocate might interview the surgeon(s) who have been suggested. Also, the advocate might be able to ask questions of the physicians and other medical personnel that the patient, in his or her confusion, might not be able to think of. Having an advocate helps the patient understand what is involved and retain a sense of choice and control, which impacts positively upon his or her recovery.

In addition, the patient should be sure that his or her wishes concerning prolonging life and medical intervention are known and clearly understood by both the family and the medical staff. If there is time, the best thing to do is to put it in writing. Most hospitals have the necessary living will and other forms.

Finally, at the end of the next chapter (page 81) there are suggestions for what the patient might do in the short time before surgery to prepare mentally and psychologically for the surgery and the subsequent healing process.

S UGGESTED   R EADING

Fontana, A. F., R. D. Kerns, R. L. Rosenberg, and K. L. Colonese. 1989. Support, stress, and recovery from coronary heart disease: A longitudinal causal model. *Health Psychology* 8: 175–193.

Kulik, J. A., and H. I. M. Mahler. 1989. Social support and recovery from surgery. *Health Psychology* 8: 221–238.

Pell, A. R. 1991. *Diagnosing Your Doctor.* Minneapolis, MN: DCI Publishing.

Silver, N. 1990. Off the pedestal. *San Francisco Chronicle,* Nov. 27, pp. B3–B4.

Tanne, J. H. 1990. How to judge a doctor. *San Francisco Chronicle,* Nov. 27, p. B4.

THREE

· · · · · · · · · · ·

PREPARING YOUR MIND AND
YOUR EMOTIONS FOR
SURGERY

T his chapter addresses some of the major psychological issues involved in bypass surgery and suggests several techniques you might employ in preparing for surgery as well as for life afterward. Again, I have assumed that you will have sufficient time to prepare for the surgery. Should this not be the case and you face emergency surgery, turn to page 81 for some suggestions about what you might do to prepare your mind and your emotions for the surgery. Also, remember that when there is limited time much of the psychological work suggested here can be accomplished after the operation.

COGNITIVE APPROACHES

When we are cognizant of something, we are *aware* or *knowing* of it. Cognitive approaches to heart bypass surgery are those that require you to be aware of and understand the surgery itself. Some cognitive procedures require the manipulation of thoughts. For example, *thought stopping* and *distracting* are simple procedures in which we deliberately stop our thought processes and shift our attention away from distressing thoughts to more neutral or calming ones.

Perhaps the most powerful technique for preparing for your surgery is information-gathering, which is a widely acknowledged major coping strategy. Information-gathering tends to accomplish two goals; it helps us contain our anxieties and it gives us an internal sense of control. Frequently, because you will have to sign an informed-consent form before surgery, you will receive verbal and written information from the hospital and/or surgeon about the procedures and some of the hospital routines. In addition, you can glean information through your own efforts by reading books, articles, interviewing others, etc.

Understanding the surgical procedure and the pre- and post-surgical process in general terms is helpful for most people preparing for bypass surgery. The known is less terrifying than the unknown. Thus, being informed about the specifics of what the surgeon will do, and of the overall goal of the surgery, is important in containing your anxiety. Research suggests that such knowledge may be helpful in promoting recovery. The underlying idea is that knowledge forewarns one, and prepares the patient to cope with both the physical and mental stresses of surgery and recovery.

Health psychologist Irving Janis coined the term "stress inoculation" to describe the process of providing preparatory forewarnings and information about impending surgical procedures and/or crises. Such preparatory information functions like an antigen, which induces the formation of disease-fighting antibodies. In other words, an individual who is prepared for difficulties and problems in the near future has an opportunity to anticipate, to start the psychological work, and to make the pragmatic and psychological plans that would promote effective coping. Janis and others have found that surgical patients:

> who receive information about the unpleasant consequences beforehand are less likely than those given little information to overreact to setbacks during the postoperative period. . . . [Considerable research shows] that when physicians or nurses give preoperative information about the stresses of surgery and ways of coping with those stresses, adult patients show less postoperative distress and sometimes better recovery from surgery.*

Achieving a thorough understanding of the surgery is the minimum amount of psychological preparation you ought to do. Most surgeons and/or their staff will be willing to spend as much time with you as you need, explaining what will be done in the surgery and the various hospital procedures you and your family might encounter. You might also ask if the hospital has any literature describing the surgery and/or hospital routine, or if there are books that you can obtain. On page 38 is a reading list of books and articles that explain the heart bypass operation.

When there is little time to prepare for surgery, at least make sure that you understand exactly what the surgery entails. Any further psychological work rests on the assimilation and understanding of these basic facts.

*Irving J. Janis and Judith Rodin, in an article entitled "Attribution, Control, and Decision Making: Social Psychology and Health Care," reprinted in *Health Psychology: a Handbook: Theories, Applications and Challenges of a Psychological Approach to the Health Care System,* edited by George C. Stone, F. Cohen, and N.E. Adler (San Francisco: Jossey-Bass, Inc., Publishers, and London: Jossey-Bass Ltd., 1979).

MIND-BODY APPROACHES

Once you have an understanding and awareness of the technical aspects of bypass surgery, you can turn to the important work of preparing your mind to deal with the stresses—and opportunities—that the surgery presents. This work involves such noncognitive approaches as Progressive Relaxation, meditation, hypnosis (including self-hypnosis), visualization, massage, or one of several mind-body techniques such as yoga, the Alexander Technique, or the Feldenkrais method. All of these techniques help relax the muscles, reduce anxiety, and achieve an inner confidence and calm. In a relatively calm, relaxed state the individual often finds that the terrors and fears of anticipated events lose their potency, and the mind is freed to think more clearly and to plan ahead more effectively.

Progressive Relaxation

In preparing people for surgery, I often recommend the process called *Progressive Relaxation,* which involves focusing your attention on each small region of your body sequentially. By alternately tensing and relaxing a particular area, and by breathing deeply and slowly, you relax each part in turn until the whole body feels relaxed. Like most noncognitive procedures, relaxation seems to work best when you close your eyes, thus limiting external distraction and stimuli.

First, place yourself in a comfortable position either seated or lying down. If lying down, it is preferable to be on your back. If seated, uncross your legs and place your feet flat on the floor. Next, focus your attention on your toes, *slowly* tensing them and then relaxing them. At each relaxation, take in a deep breath and let it out *slowly.* Repeat the tense-relax process two or three times. Note in your mind how different each body part feels when it is tensed compared to when it is relaxed. Note also how *you* feel as the various body parts let go of their tension. When your toes feel relaxed, move your attention to your feet, repeating the process of first tensing and then relaxing them, breathing slowly and deeply as they relax. When your feet are relaxed, refocus your attention to your calves, repeating the tense-relax-breathe sequence, then focus in turn on your thighs, lower abdomen, upper abdomen, chest, neck, head and face, shoulders, back, buttocks, and arms, until each part of your body is relaxed. Be sure to include the region around your eyes and mouth, since many of us carry a lot of tension there. The shoulders are also a major repository of body tension for most people, and they need your comforting attention.

Meditation and Visualization

Two other techniques I find helpful in preparing people for bypass surgery are meditation and visualization. These techniques, which have been used for thousands of years as a means of gaining wisdom and understanding, are frequently used as stress management procedures because they are excellent ways to quiet the mind. Each procedure begins with finding a quiet place where you can either sit or lie down comfortably and allow your body to relax as you attend to your breathing by slowing it down and deepening it.

Meditation is aimed at refocusing the mind's usual activity. It is essentially similar to self-hypnosis or any other method of entering a trance state, or an altered state of consciousness. One enters a trance state by concentrating on some rhythmic and repetitive thought, sound, or action. Although much has been made of the "mystery" of meditative concentration and the tremendous powers it supposedly brings to its practitioners, you need not believe any of this to derive mental and physical benefits from the process. Meditation can be used effectively to lower blood pressure and to promote health simply by helping you relax and reduce the tension stored in the body's musculature. Meditation and other trance techniques can be used productively to prepare for bypass surgery and to help rebuild your life after the operation.

There are many ways to meditate. Here is one simple technique. Prepare for meditation by using the progressive relaxation procedure described above. When you feel relaxed, focus your attention on the rhythm of your breathing. As thoughts intrude into your awareness, acknowledge them but then allow them to pass, and return your attention to the breathing. Some people find that the meditative process is facilitated when they repeat a short phrase or word over and over again (generally in rhythm with their breathing). This is often referred to as saying a "mantra." Some individuals focus their awareness in their "mind's eye," a spot in space just in front of and a few inches above their forehead. This spot often appears to them as a bright white light.

Another way to enter a meditative state is through slow stretching exercises. Many persons who exercise regularly, employ stretching techniques to prepare their muscles for the strenuous workout they will receive during the course of the exercise. Stretching is also used in the "cool-down" after the exercise is done. When the latter stretching movements are slowed down, they often help the person achieve a meditative or trance state. Some individuals use the movements of yoga or tai chi chuan for such purposes, although significantly slowing down almost any movement would work just as well.

Meditation can be done at anytime and anywhere. As with most activities, regular practice makes meditation easier to do and the trance state easier to achieve. With practice, one might meditate while exercising or carrying out some other patterned, routine action. For example, working out on a stationary exercise bicycle is a perfect time to meditate. With practice, even a short meditation of less than a minute may have positive effects for the individual.

Using Visualization to Prepare for Bypass Surgery

Perhaps the most powerful technique to use in preparing for surgery is to set time aside on a regular basis to visualize or image the surgical procedures from start to finish. This is best accomplished in a quiet place like a dimly lit room where distractions can be kept to a minimum and where you feel secure and comfortable. Begin first by relaxing, perhaps by using the Progressive Relaxation procedure.

Visualization, or imagery, is the process of deliberately forming mental pictures—that is, visual images in your mind—of a scene or occurrence. Have you ever watched the Olympic gold medalist Carl Lewis prepare for a long jump? He frequently mouths words to himself as he puts his body through some of the motions (in an abbreviated form) he will use in the forthcoming jump. In short, he is visualizing, and rehearsing in his mind, the entire jump, from beginning to end, saying things to himself, in conjunction with each anticipated movement, that encourage and assist him to accomplish the feat. He is using the process of imagery in combination with his cognitive understanding to prepare for successful action. This is what makes him a champion.

Each of us has the capacity to use our mind in that way. The late pianist Walter Gieseking was said to have such powers of imagination that he seldom practiced the difficult pieces he played in recital, preferring instead to spend most of his time in mental concentration, visualizing the playing, the finger positions, the sequence, and the pressure on the keys. Fortunately, in preparing for bypass surgery one does not need to have such talents or to go that far in the imagery process to obtain positive results.

To help achieve a positive outcome, in visualizing bypass surgery, two goals should be kept in mind: *owning the surgery* and *welcoming it*—that is, thinking of it in positive terms rather than as an assault on your body.

To make the surgery your own, it is necessary to *take responsibility for the decision* to have the surgery. Physicians may recommend the procedure, but the ultimate decision to proceed is the patient's, and it should be an active rather than a passive decision. You might think of yourself as being either an active participant or a passive spectator to an event that has profound implications for your life. If you are consciously aware, the surgery cannot be forced on you. If you have the surgery, it is because you have deliberately chosen to do so.

If you accept responsibility for the surgical decision, it becomes possible to view the surgeon as your personal instrument in achieving the goal of restoring health. The surgeon thus becomes a partner and a guide in making you whole again—helping you re-find a life path that has temporarily become obscured.

When you "choose" surgery because you feel that there is no other choice, or out of necessity or fear, you are acting out of desperation and helplessness. The surgeon in such circumstances is seen as a saviour rather than as a partner, and you perceive yourself as being powerless. Powerlessness promotes passivity. Actively choosing to take responsibility for the surgical decision makes the surgery (and its outcome) your own, which leads to involvement in active decision-making later on.

Once you have made the surgery your own, you need to deal

with the surgery as a welcomed process rather than as an assault or physical violation of your body. Because the chest is opened and the heart tampered with, it is easy to view the surgery as an invasion. Some physicians and other medical personnel actually describe it in just that way. It's important, therefore, to adopt a different viewpoint, one that is positive, constructive, and focused on the goal of surgery, which is to restore you to health. One powerful technique is to view the physical intrusion as a means to an end, and to view the surgeon as a welcome guest—a repair person of the highest order, someone you will invite inside your body to put things right.

If you perceive of the surgery as an assault, the body will protect itself in advance, and stay in that protective place for a longer period of time afterward, thus retarding the healing and recovery processes. If, on the other hand, you can put your mind and body in a more receptive mode, receptive of the cutting, opening, and stitching, and in full understanding that there will be discomfort and pain, then healing and recovery is already underway even before the surgical procedures are over.

At issue is whether you view the surgery with resentment or with acceptance and welcome. Whichever attitude you choose will ultimately affect how your body responds before, during, and after surgery. Increasing evidence suggests that recovery and healing are facilitated by the positive presurgical attitude of patients.

Suggested Exercises for Visualization and Meditation

Owning the Surgery. One visualization that might help you own the surgery is to think of what is happening as a personal journey. During this journey you have come to a stream that cannot be forded, but which you must get across in order to reach your destination. The only conveyance is a ferry and the surgeon is the captain of the ferry. The captain and crew will take you across the stream to the other side where you will be able to continue onward toward your goal. You willingly pay the fare and climb aboard. Such images reinforce the fact that you are the one who makes the decisions about your health and about the action you will take to maintain and improve it.

Welcoming the Surgery. To help yourself welcome the surgery, imagine that the surgeon is a new friend you have just made, someone with whom you want to share an important part of your life. You extend an invitation for the surgeon to enter your home (your body) as an honored guest. Imagine that you are opening your heart to him or her in friendship and goodwill. For some individuals, the image of an accompanying lavish banquet you have set out seems to bring pleasure. For other individuals, the image of the guest arriving and helping you repair some part of the home plumbing brings a sense of satisfaction (and sometimes amusement) and underscores the sense of amity and partnership.

Using Commercial Audiotapes. Generic imagery and meditation audiotapes are readily available on the market to help you establish a positive mindset for surgery. These tapes tend to focus on the issues of relaxation, the belief in a positive outcome, and the mobilization of your inner healing forces to speed the recovery process. One difficulty I find with these tapes is that they tend to promote passivity rather than encourage the patient to remain active in exploring his or her inner realms and in diving deeper within the psyche to find guidance and courage. Also, the audiotapes can deal only with the general case, not with the specific issues each individual brings to the situation.

Visualizing the Surgical Procedure. Visualizing or imagining the surgical procedure might be split up into smaller segments such as (1) going to the hospital, (2) spending the first day in the hospital, (3) prepping on the day of surgery and being wheeled to the operating room, (4) coming through the surgery itself, (5) waking up and returning to life, (6) the healing process. Try spending fifteen to twenty minutes each day, or twice a day, visualizing one of these small segments. Here are some guidelines to help you "see" each part of the process.

Either sitting comfortably or lying down, begin to see yourself on the way to the hospital and then being admitted for surgery. Paint as many details as you can. Mentally rehearse getting into your car, pulling out of the driveway, and driving to the hospital. Perhaps a significant other is at your side or is driving the vehicle. Imagine yourself arriving at the hospital, parking the car, walking into the hospital to the information desk or to the office where the registration procedures will be done. Try to imagine these procedures. It is likely that after the paperwork is out of the way you will be placed in a wheelchair and escorted to a nursing station, and to the room that will be your home for a day or so. Imagine the room, the bed, the atmosphere. Imagine a nurse welcoming you, and handing you a hospital gown to change into. Picture yourself changing into the gown.

More than likely you have never been to the hospital where the surgery will be done so you will have to base your imagery and rehearsal efforts on experiences gained from watching TV or from visiting friends in other hospitals. Also, your surgeon and his or her staff may give you some information about the hospital and the procedures you might expect to encounter on your day of admission. Use all these memories and materials to add detail to your mental picture. As you rehearse these simple steps you will most likely feel a greater sense of security and control over the unknown.

On the day you are admitted to the hospital, you will probably meet a number of different professionals, including the anesthesiologist and the other members of the surgical team. You will probably be X-rayed, undergo an electrocardiogram, have blood drawn, and receive a thorough physical examination. A physical or exercise therapist, nutritionist, respiration therapist, and others will come by to talk to you and fill in some of the details of the postsurgical period. Continue your visualization by imagining one or two of these various professionals and see yourself interacting with them. Look forward to meeting these individuals, because they are on your side and want you to come through the surgery with flying colors.

As you go to sleep the night before the surgery, you will probably be given some medication to help you relax and sleep. When you wake you will probably shower and be prepared for the actual surgery. You may be given more medication at this point so that your memory of the events to follow may be difficult to retrieve after the fact.

Allow yourself in imagination to see yourself on a gurney (a stretcher on wheels) being wheeled to the operating room. Be aware that by that time you will probably be in an anesthetically induced sleep or will be so drowsy that you have no real-time memory of the event. Picture yourself being moved carefully onto the operating table and then having the surgical team place hypodermic needles into your arms and neck. Imagine the surgical team readying itself to perform the surgery.

As I imagined these events in my own preparation for surgery, I kept giving myself the message that, *"Everything is going OK. Everything will be OK."* I saw myself at peace, secure. I found it helpful to keep repeating to myself, "The team knows its job; *everything is going to be OK.*"

In imagination, I saw myself during the operation, listening to the muffled voices around me, like listening to music from afar. Their voices sounded friendly, matter of fact, calm—*everything was going to be OK.* I saw myself drift into a deep, restorative, untroubled, peaceful sleep. Imagine that the operation is over and you have come through it successfully. Picture yourself, placed again on a gurney, being wheeled to and placed on a bed in the recovery room or in the intensive care unit.

Now imagine yourself in the immediate postsurgical period, lying in bed in the intensive care unit. Consciousness may return as suddenly as if a switch had been thrown. You will probably not experience any pain since you will most likely have received pain medication. You will not be alone; someone—probably a nurse—will be there attending and watching you. You will become aware of the fact that you cannot speak since a tube has been put in place in your mouth and trachea. This tube is connected to a respirator and as soon as you can breathe on your own it will be removed. Because of the pain medication you received and because the gag reflex stops after a certain amount of time, you will probably not be discomforted by the tracheal tube. Now let your mental picture advance a day or so and imagine yourself walking slowly down the hospital corridor. You are on the road to recovery.

PROMOTING SURVIVAL

One fear that many persons have in preparing for bypass surgery is that of dying. As they begin to imagine themselves in the operating room, thoughts of a deep sleep inevitably lead to thoughts of how easy it would be just to slip away into the endless night, painlessly. How tempting. The person would be medicated and wouldn't feel anything. No fear, no angst, no pain. If one must die, what better way than that?

These thoughts are fueled by several factors. First, although the odds are in the patient's favor, the procedure is not risk-free. Second, many of us either know or have heard of someone who did not survive bypass surgery. In my case, my daughter-in-law's father, Bill, had died in just this way some three years earlier and that tragic event was still fresh in our memory. The unspoken feeling we all had was that he had given up on life and, perhaps, welcomed death.

In preparing for surgery, it is advisable that you go deep inside yourself to question whether or not you are committed to life or whether on some level you have resigned yourself to the idea that life is over anyway. No one knows for sure whether or not one can bring about one's death merely by wishing it—or, to put it another way, by not wishing for life. But determination and willpower do have an impact on our lives. Survivors of concentration camp experiences report that many individuals gave up on life and died shortly thereafter, whereas others, through sheer determination, continued to hang on day by day and eventually survived their horrendous ordeal.

A person's beliefs do influence how he or she approaches life tasks. If you deeply believe that you will survive major surgery because of a commitment to continue living, the chances are good that your "decision" will mobilize psychological and physiological mechanisms that can assist your body to cope with the surgery and that can promote recovery and survival.

Avoiding thinking about the possibility of death neither promotes survival nor allows you or your family to face and prepare for the realistic, although unlikely, possibility that you will not make it through. On the contrary: Thinking about and planning for realistic possibilities, even ones with low likelihood, has been shown over and over again to improve the later coping capacities of individuals and families.

Psychologically, an inner calm occurs when we know that things in our lives are in place. Either consciously or unconsciously we know when our personal affairs are in disarray and not attended to properly. On some level we know, and that knowledge affects how we feel, how high our anxiety levels will be, and how much confidence we display. No one undergoing bypass surgery wants to think about not surviving, but you should not delude yourself that death is not a possibility. Talking about it and planning for it will help you and your family know that things are in place.

When I was struggling with the issue of whether or not I wanted to survive the surgery, a mantra-like word came to me during a meditation. The word was *live*. This simple word had enormous psychological power to calm the doubts, turmoil, and angst that had marked the weeks prior to the decision to proceed with the surgery, and provided the courage and strength to move forward toward the day of the operation.

In addition to the preparations I was making on my own, my wife was helping me through suggestions and also trance work. One of the most important suggestions she made was to think about going into surgery with a protector, like a guardian angel. She suggested a positive figure, my father-in-law, who, like my father, had died of a heart attack, but unlike him had lived an active, positive life up until the end. He would be with me in spirit during the surgery to watch over and protect me. Other individuals often select religious figures to be with them during the surgery.

In retrospect, this seems like such a childlike strategy for dealing with impending stress. But at the time, there is something powerfully appropriate, pleasing, and comforting in thinking and believing in this childlike way. After all, surgery requires that you give up adult controls and defenses and, if that is the case, what is wrong with adopting the defenses that worked earlier in life? If the thought that guardian angels will watch over you brings comfort and encourages you to move forward without paralyzing fear, then by all means get yourself a guardian angel!

INVOLVING YOUR SPOUSE OR SIGNIFICANT OTHER

If you have a significant other in your life, involve him or her in your preparations for surgery. It reinforces the feeling that you are not alone. One way your partner might help you (and themselves in the process) is by setting aside an hour or so each day before the surgery for you to talk intimately with one another. He or she might also assist you to relax and to meditate. For example, he/she might give you a gentle massage, particularly on or around your shoulders, back, and chest, and with soothing, encouraging, reassuring words help you get in touch with your feelings and thoughts.

I had the good fortune of having a wife who is also a clinical psychologist and who could use hypnosis to prepare me for the surgery. Fortunately, your spouse or significant other does not need such specialized training to apply the mind-body techniques discussed here. The ability to help you relax and to experience inner calm either through gentle words and/or a comforting touch is all that's needed.

More about the spouse's role in preparing for surgery can be found in Chapter 6.

RESOLVING ISSUES FROM THE PAST

Inevitably as you prepare for the surgery, personal issues out of the past tend to emerge. For example, the necessity of bypass surgery brought me in touch with my long-deceased father. He had angina problems for a good part of his adult life and it debilitated him. His life was restricted and he went through it mostly as an invalid. In health and illness my father was my primary male adult model and his influence on my thinking and behavior was profound. I had had difficulty using him as a positive model for either how he lived or how he died. My adolescence and much of my adult life was taken up in differentiating myself from him. In many ways, I had succeeded in being different from him, but there was a significant part of him that remained in me, locked in my chest around my heart, as if he were an unbidden guest. By focusing on my heart and the symbolic fact that bypass surgery would "free" my heart to live again, I was able to make peace with my father and our relationship—to let go and free myself of certain memories and burdens.

Invariably we all incorporate aspects of our parents' personalities within ourselves whether we want to or not since they are our initial life models. Psychologists speak of such incorporations as "introjects." They are perpetually with us, and the more honest we are with ourselves, the more we see them, for better or worse, in the way we think, relate, and act. Describing his own bypass experience in *The New York Times Magazine* (December 30, 1990; pages 17–22) novelist Philip Roth wrote:

> I realized that never had I been more at one with my father than I was at that moment: not since college, when I used to secretly imagine him in class with me . . . had our lives been, if not identical, so inter-meshed and spookily interchangeable.

For some individuals there is an awareness of an association between a specific body part and the parental introject. In my case, I experienced my father as being lodged in my chest near my heart. This realization occurred during a massage in which thoughts of my father arose as my chest was gently touched.

In preparing for the bypass surgery, my attention was naturally centered on this part of my body and all the associations that went with it. It became evident that one of my major psychological tasks was to rid myself of this introject or at least remove its power over my behavior. Psychologically, this meant I had to separate myself sufficiently so that my life script became my own rather than my father's. He had lived his life; I had to live mine. He had lived a life of debilitation whereas I wished to live a life of health and vitality.

In a meditation it became clear to me that my father was not a ghost inside of me; he didn't even want to be there. Rather, I discovered that *I* was holding on to *him*. It was time to let go.

In the week prior to the surgery I used the opportunity to meditate and engage in an inner dialogue with my father and, so to speak, prepare him for his exit and for my taking over my own chest and heart, my own life. It was our ultimate separation and differentiation. Thus, in my inward preparations for surgery, I imagined myself opened up and my father's "soul" liberated, floating away to its own place of rest in the universe. He was pleased to be freed and to see his son take over his own life. On a not-too-profound level, it was another way of saying to myself that I wanted to live a healthy, full life, not the life of debilitation and limitation that angina and heart disease had imposed on my father.

PREPARATION FOR HEALING

Just as it is important to prepare yourself psychologically for the surgery, so you also need to prepare for the healing process afterward. Some individuals find it helpful before surgery to image or meditate on the new blood vessels they will receive in the course of surgery and to picture them as open and healthy, allowing the nourishing blood to flow through them effortlessly. Others focus their attention on the scar that will result from opening the chest wall and picture their cells actively working together to heal the injuries left by the surgery. Some individuals tend to get in touch, in meditation, with various body parts and to ask these parts what it is they need or what message they have to give. This is a meditation or visualization exercise in which you engage in an inner dialogue with your body or body parts, giving the part a voice to instruct or to inform the mind. When I engaged in this exercise, I received a guiding word to help me in moments of anxiety, a simple, encouraging, mantra-like statement: the word *heal*. The word had enormous power, allowing me to enter meditative states more easily and more deeply and to emerge from such states in greater peace. I was aware that the word *health* also contained the message "heal," and so the concepts became fused.

One site often forgotten in this preparatory work is the leg from which a vein will probably be removed during the surgery and used as a bypass graft. The scar left on the leg sometimes heals quickly, but for some that scar may become more problematic than the rest of the surgery. I advise that some effort be made to guide/instruct your leg to create new circulation routes, once the vein is gone, and to cooperate in your process of healing.

Some centers at which bypass surgery is done now offer patients the option of listening to music of their choice during surgery. This has a certain attractiveness since it now seems that even under anesthesia the patient is not entirely oblivious to what is going on. Listening to music might help to distract you from the background noise and chatter usually going on in the operating room during surgery. An alternative, possibly more active, approach is to take on a productive task during this "out" period. For example, in her preparatory work Hilda suggested that I use the time under anesthesia to allow my mind to wander into the unknown, to rendezvous with whomever or whatever I chose, and to acquire whatever wisdom I could. She called this "entering the realm of the gods." It was left up to me to entertain whatever fantasy, desire, wish, or curiosity I cared to during this somnolence and to return to consciousness with the knowledge and insights I had acquired on my journey to put to use in the recovery period.

THE FAMILY'S CONTRIBUTION

Up until this point, we have concentrated on the things that you, the patient, can do to prepare for surgery. But chances are you are not alone in facing this ordeal. Generally there is a mate, family, and/or group of friends who participate in the process of preparation. And their actions can either facilitate or impede your own preparations. The attitudes and anxieties of family and friends can play a major role in determining the outcome of your surgery, so it makes good sense for you to shape those attitudes and allay those anxieties as much as possible.

One family I worked with tended to handle their anxieties ineffectively. Whenever any family event occurred that aroused anxiety (and this might include funerals, weddings, and the like, as well as illnesses) the various family members began to become demanding of one another. Frequently, arguments broke out over trivial things, and whatever joy individuals might feel on happy occasions tended to be dissipated. If there was sorrow or grief in the occasion, this was often magnified and individual feelings could not be shared with the family as a whole. Interactions between family members often left one or more persons unhappy, unsatisfied, and frustrated.

Jack, the patriarch of the family, had to undergo some of the medical procedures such as angiography leading up to bypass surgery. This necessity aroused enormous anxiety among the various family members, and Jack's wife, Mary, spent almost all her emotional energy trying to placate their children who, predictably, became overly demanding of attention. For example, all the children decided separately to visit their parents with their young children the week of the angiogram. The visits brought multiple complications about the logistics of being picked up from airports, transportation problems, babysitting, and so on, all of which added to Jack's preprocedural anxiety. By concentrating on the logistical problems, Mary contained her own anxiety about what her husband was going through. But, on the other hand, she could not provide the attention and protection Jack needed, nor could she carry out her own psychological preparations. The situation was one in which there was enormous concern for what was happening to Jack and for Jack himself. However, because of the difficulty in containing anxiety, no deep psychological work was possible. It did not seem to occur to anyone that their father might need some peace and quiet at that time rather than the tumult family visits usually brought.

At the other extreme are Frank and Joan. Frank required bypass surgery, and his grown children flew in from the east coast to be with their parents during the week in which Frank would be in the hospital. Joan, in contrast to Mary above, was overly protective of her husband to the point that she did not allow anyone outside the nuclear family to visit him before or after the surgery. Friends who wished to come to the hospital were dissuaded from doing so, which cut Frank off from his usual social interactions and probably interfered with a rapid return to normal functioning.

Visits by friends and relatives, if they are part of your usual routine, are important in the postsurgical period. Such visits generally require you to mobilize your energies to be presentable to others, just as you would do in normal times. Psychologically, you have the opportunity to practice being healthy and normal even though you are still recuperating from the surgery. Thus, although it may be tiring for you, it may also feel like a triumph to receive and "entertain" visitors.

Some patients handle their anxieties by denying that they are anxious. Generally, their significant others balance the universe by being anxious for both of them. Little attention is given by the medical system to the needs of significant others in such situations and not inconsiderable suffering occurs because almost all attention is focused on the needs of the patient rather than on those of both partners. The nonsurgical partner often bears an unusually heavy burden, which may take a long time to recover from and to resolve. Bypass surgery also often has an impact on the patient's children. It not only brings them closer to their parents' mortality but also makes them aware of their own finiteness.

For some adult children with conflicts or difficulties, let us say in the area of relationships or marriage, the parent's surgery sometimes promotes a maturation that might not otherwise occur at this period of their lives. In interviews with individuals who underwent surgery, several mentioned that their adult children had effected major life changes (getting married, for example) soon after the surgery. Others reported a deepening of their relations with their children and the resolution of long-standing conflicts. It is almost as if everyone becomes aware of the pettiness of some problems and the fact that the clock of life is ticking and there isn't too much time left.

IN CASE OF EMERGENCY BYPASS SURGERY

1. To the extent that you can, understand in general terms what the procedures will be during and after the surgery; if you need help, ask the nurse or doctor to provide an advocate.

2. If time permits, visualize the procedures in your mind.

3. If you can, visualize yourself being operated on; remind yourself that the professionals around you know their jobs and all you have to do at this point is to cooperate.

4. Remember that your chances of survival are generally high.

5. Visualize yourself waking up after the surgery; someone will be with you and will help orient you; remember, you will not be alone.

6. Remind yourself that when you have recovered from the surgery you will have the time to organize all the things left undone.

7. Remind yourself that your friends and loved ones are rooting for you, that they care about and love you; tell them that you care about and love them.

8. Don't be ashamed of how afraid you might feel; talk about it to anyone near you; most people will understand.

9. Remember that you have faced adversity in the past and come through. Have courage; you can do it again.

Four

· · · · · · · · · · ·

HEART BYPASS: A PERSONAL
EXPERIENCE

This chapter describes a typical first day in the hospital for the bypass patient, and what is likely to happen in the immediate postsurgical period. In addition to an overview of hospital routine, the chapter contains entries from two diaries—those of a heart bypass patient *and* his wife. Having this dual perspective allows you to see what was happening to the patient at all times during the surgery, even when he was under the influence of anesthesia, pain killers, and other medications. It also enables you to see the impact that bypass surgery has on the patient's family, especially in the early stages of recuperation.

WHAT TO EXPECT ON YOUR FIRST DAY IN THE HOSPITAL

Many hospitals require that you check in a day or so before surgery to receive some orientation and for various laboratory tests and procedures. It's also likely that you will receive a thorough medical examination so that the surgeons will not have any surprises during the surgery.

If you have not already met the surgical team, this generally is the time that various team members come by to introduce themselves, describe their respective roles, and answer questions. Besides the surgeons, a key member of the surgical team is the anesthesiologist, who often will describe the pharmaceuticals that will be used and their effects during and after the surgery. Generally, the anesthetics used during bypass surgery leave the patient with retrograde amnesia—that is, with no memory of the immediate presurgical or surgical periods.

Other professionals might come by to talk to you as well. One is the respiration therapist, who is likely to give you a device, an incentive spirometer, that will be a constant companion in the postsurgical period. It may consist of a plastic graduated cylinder inside of which is a plastic ball. A flexible hose with an attached mouthpiece allows you to take a deep breath and see the ball rise in the cylinder. The height to which the ball rises depends on the depth of the inhalation. The more air you draw in, the higher the ball goes. Following the surgery you use this device to increase the depth of your breathing, which is essential to recovering full lung function.

Generally, the day ends with your being given a Fleet enema.

A PATIENT'S DIARY (MY OWN)

Early Tuesday morning, when it was still dark outside, I was awakened and given some special brown soap with which to shower. I was also given some pills to take, and the last thing I clearly remember before the surgery was having a discussion with a nurse about how peculiar it felt to feel simultaneously afraid and calm. Apparently, shortly after the shower I was helped on to a gurney and taken to the operating room, where the hair on my chest, pubic region, and left leg were shaved. I say apparently because I have no memory of it whatsoever. My family reported to me afterward that they had been with me during some of the period just prior to my being wheeled in for surgery, that I had engaged in conversation with them, and had told them more or less the same thing I had said to the nurse, that I loved them, etc. I have no memory of these events or conversations. I'll just take their word for it. It feels right.

They also told me that they had seen me being wheeled out from the operating room after the surgery was over and that later on they had been with me, talked to me (I apparently didn't answer), held my hand, and so on. At one point, someone asked me to squeeze their hand and I was told that I did so. My wife also told me later on that I had responded with a hand squeeze when she had visited me Tuesday evening, either in response to something she had said or more likely to her holding and squeezing my hand. These memories remain indistinct as if there are some memory traces there that I cannot fully retrieve.

Regaining Consciousness

When I first became conscious, I was aware of being confused by the sights and sounds around me. I recall thinking, "Where am I? Is the surgery over? What time is it?" My mind felt alert and yet at the same time it all felt like a dream. I felt no pain. In fact, my body felt full of energy. It was like suddenly waking from a long, restful nap.

There was a nurse at my bedside and I tried to talk but was unable to make more than some grunting sounds. I became aware of the tube in my mouth and remembered thinking, "Well, I guess the surgery is over." But, somehow I wasn't sure. Maybe the surgery hadn't been done yet. Perhaps the tube had been inserted in preparation for the surgery. I needed to hear someone say, "The surgery is over and everything's OK." Perhaps they did say this and it didn't register.

I wasn't frightened. If anything, I was intensely curious—like a newborn baby first opening its eyes and wondering, "Where am I?" "Where is this?" "Who are these people?" "What is this all about?"

What day was it? I tried to ask the nurse and she misinterpreted my grunts to mean that I was in pain. I recall she said that I had received pain medication recently and that she couldn't give me any more at that time. I wasn't the least bit interested in medication. I wanted to know what day it was. The need to communicate with her became intense and I made signs to her to bring me something to write on and something to write with. It took her a while to catch on and until she did I began to feel agitated out of frustration. At the same time I remember feeling amused at the situation, as if there was a part of me delightfully impish and easily tickled by what seemed silly. When she brought a pencil and paper I attempted to write the questions, "What time is it and what day is it"? but as I wrote the pencil angled down the page in an unintelligible scrawl. I remember feeling a sense of despair when I realized that no one could possibly read my scribblings. Something within me snapped and I became even more determined to communicate. I tore off the top sheet of paper and on the next sheet in large letters wrote, "What DAY"? The nurse could read it, but, unfortunately, she could not understand the question's meaning. She responded, "Yes, it's daytime." If I could have hit the ceiling I would have. I became even more insistent and shaking my head and grunting as loud as I could, attempted to shout, "Damn it, what day of the week is it?" And again, there was a part of me just laughing at the humor of the situation. Finally, the nursing supervisor arrived and answered my question. She understood perfectly what I needed. "It's Wednesday," she told me. My whole body relaxed and for the first time in what felt like hours, I felt at peace. It was Wednesday and my surgery had been scheduled for Tuesday. That meant that I was on the other side of the surgery. It was over. I was alive. I had made it. Everything was going to be OK. It turned out that all of these events had transpired in the early morning hours. I had slept through all of Tuesday following the surgery. I was in the Coronary Intensive Care Unit, where my heartbeat, blood pressure, and other vital functions were continuously monitored by the machinery around me.

I gradually became aware of the tubes coming out of my lower chest, the one taped to my face and inserted into my nose supplying me with oxygen, and the Foley catheter in place for drainage of my bladder. I was told later that I had also had tubes coming out of my neck, but these had been removed by the time I became conscious. There was an IV in place in my left hand.

The removal of each tube represented a step forward toward recuperation. The first step was to determine whether or not I could breathe on my own. This was done by turning off the breathing machinery and watching how I managed on my own. When it was certain I was breathing just fine without the assistance of outside machinery, the tracheal tube was pulled out. It was a glorious release; I was able to talk again. This was accomplished by Wednesday morning, less than twenty-four hours after surgery. Before the day was over, the Foley catheter was removed and I was able to pass water on my own. I was also helped up out of bed and took my first steps.

The Rest of the Hospital Stay

On the following day, one of the chest tubes was taken out, and, with assistance from a nurse and my wife, I walked slowly down the corridor to a new room in the telemetry unit. Whereas in intensive care I had twenty-four-hour, one-on-one direct monitoring of all functions, in the telemetry unit I was connected to a monitor in the nursing station and my functions were monitored indirectly. It was like graduating from primary school to secondary school.

On Friday the last chest tube was taken out and, frankly, this was about the most painful experience I ever had. It had all the features of a combination toothache/smacking your thumb with a hammer experience. Although the locus of the experience is pretty small, your whole body reacts and it takes your breath away. Fortunately, the pain subsides and you become aware that another major step toward discharge from the hospital has been achieved.

I wish that the physician who pulled the tube out had given me a bit more warning and sent my family out of the room so that I could have given full reign to the scream I felt I had to suppress in order not to frighten my little granddaughter who was in the room at the time. Fortunately, my son was with me holding my hand at the time. I could see by the look on his face how shaken he was from the experience.

Each day, as I improved and became stronger, I walked around the corridors of the unit either with my wife or, if she was not there, on my own. I found that I had little appetite for the food that was brought to me. True, it wasn't exactly gourmet cuisine. But, even if it had been I don't think I could have eaten it. In fact, I seemed to be attracted to rather bland foods—a baked potato, a little Jell-o, those kinds of things. The food was entirely unsalted because, I was told, my salt intake had to be restricted to help reduce the edema, swelling, in my leg.

My poor leg. I had a surgical scar up the length of my left calf and almost halfway up my thigh. The leg was swollen to almost double its normal size. Because a large vein had been removed from the leg, the circulatory system there was not up to snuff and as a result fluid was collecting in the intercellular spaces causing swelling. Normally, such fluid is drained off via the venous system. Until a new collateral system of veins developed in the leg, there would be problems with edema.

Over the weekend I moved once again, this time to a regular room similar to the one I had when I was admitted. Time passed in an orderly sort of way. I had my walking to do several times a day. It was a great way to keep from getting bored. Whenever I felt tired, I usually sat in a chair with my leg elevated and listened to music or books on tape. Every hour or two I did my breathing exercises. This consisted of placing into my mouth the mouthpiece of a tube attached to a cylinder-like contraption in which a plastic ball was situated, and inhaling with as much gusto as possible. To the extent that the inhalation was good, the plastic ball would rise in the cylinder, which was calibrated on the outside. It became a game to see how high I could make the ball go. Sometimes I would get it to go almost halfway up the cylinder. Such exercises are crucial for helping the lungs return to normal functioning and for staying clear of secretions and mucus, which, if allowed to build up, might result in pneumonia.

Then there were the light stretching exercises, taught to me by the physical therapist, that needed to be done several times a day. Generally, my temperature and blood pressure would be taken at regular intervals during the course of a day and invariably a cardiologist would stop by each day to listen to my heart and lungs, and one of the surgeons would come by to look me over. These activities plus a few visitors kept me occupied and focused on the work of healing.

Overall, with the exception of a few brief moments, I experienced little pain during the final few days in the hospital. The feelings I had vacillated between ones of fatigue, with a desire to sleep, and those of exaltation and pride when I thought about the rapidity of my recovery. My body felt stiff as if I were muscle-bound, and when I walked about the corridors, my step was slow. I knew my body had been through a horrendous experience and needed attention and time to heal. At the same time, it felt different and somewhat strange and unfamiliar. I was aware of how close to the surface my emotions—especially those associated with warmth and affection—seemed to be. It didn't take much to bring tears to my eyes. But these were not tears of sadness or of pain, but rather ones of joy and thankfulness to be alive.

A SPOUSE'S DIARY (MY WIFE'S)

It's Monday, early afternoon, and Seymour is propped up in his hospital bed awaiting the arrival of the kids. His private room is bright and airy, tastefully decorated, and faces green hills and a blue sky. It reminds me more of a hotel room than of the stereotypic cold and sterile hospital room. When our children arrive with our granddaughter, it begins to resemble a party.

Seymour's mood is incredibly upbeat. He's enjoying all this attention. Most important, he's overjoyed to have his beloved granddaughter snuggling into him in the hospital bed. They are totally absorbed in each other, exchanging loving and affectionate glances. We all stand back and marvel at the scene. Neither one of them expresses any concern, fear, anxiety, or surprise at the setting. It is as if their souls are in communion with one another and the impending danger doesn't exist. Watching them together, I understand why it was so essential for her to be present. She represents the future, the potentiality for all possibility, the openness of tomorrow. By identifying with her, Seymour is also identifying with the future and all it holds for him. This little soul is taking him along into the future and he is a most willing passenger.

I watch our sons, watching their father. Here was a man that they had hardly seen in the past. They had known his serious, hardworking, worried side. Now they were witnessing his playful, childlike, optimistic, and believing side. His joy spread and enveloped us. There was no denying the seriousness of the situation, but it was coupled with the buoyancy of the moment and the faith that if anyone could pull off this operation, it's their father.

In the late afternoon, the children departed and Seymour and I found ourselves alone in the twilight of the day. The mood became more sober but not somber. It was a good time for us to repeat the meditative exercises we had been doing all the past week. Seymour easily, eagerly, went into a trance in which he visualized the surgery and my father's watchful presence protecting his body while his soul soared to unknown realms. He imagined his quest for knowledge in that place and the release from his own father's grip in the process. We envisioned his journey back and the reunion with his body as well as the return to those who love him. Finally, we envisioned his natural capacity to activate all his healing forces in the service of a full and speedy recovery.

Then it was time to leave and it was difficult to say good night, to walk out of his hospital room and separate after having been so close over the past several weeks. But now our journeys parted. I could not accompany him. As much as I willed myself to image his passage through the ordeal of surgery, I could not enter it with him. It was his alone.

It was not fear that motivated me to desire to stay united, but rather an awareness of our essential, irrevocable separateness that no amount of love or attachment could bridge. The knowledge was at once exquisite and piercing. It was an experience that, regardless of the outcome of the surgery, I knew I would one day repeat. It was inevitable that a time would come when we would be parted forever. It was not a new sensation. I had known it before, but its sharpness never dulled with repeated experience.

I drove home aware of my aloneness, encased in my feelings, inside a private universe. There was a sweet pleasure mingled with the pain. I felt fully alive and aware of all my sensations, emotions, and thoughts. I had removed all the usual barriers to knowing, and nothing was unacceptable to my consciousness.

At 5 A.M. the following morning, my two sons and I returned to the hospital. We wanted to be with Seymour as long as possible before he was wheeled into the surgery unit. When we arrived, he had already showered and had been given some tranquilizer. He seemed relaxed, almost buoyant. Although afterward he had no memory of the events of the morning before surgery, he was very much present and interactive.

He described his night. He had slept well, having been given a tranquilizer. In a jocular tone he described the nurse waking him up at about 4:30 for his shower and helping him in it. His usual inhibited, shy self seemed to have been peeled away. (Was this the effect of the tranquilizers or of his sense that he had nothing left to hide? I will never know for sure.) He chided me humorously for not indulging his pleasure in washing him down as the nurse had just done. I responded in kind, reminding him that there would be lots of opportunities for that in the days to come. I should have realized that he was already entering an altered level of consciousness. He seemed unaware of time, of the dawn light filtering into his room, and of the quiet in the hospital surround. He seemed pleased that we were there, as if our presence was a most natural thing. But he also seemed unaware of the events to follow.

Our older son, Elliot, stood close to him at the side of his bed and gently massaged his back, with each stroke transmitting love for his father. I watched them, aware of the significance of the son giving and of the father receiving, absorbing his son's love. Through these simple actions they were communicating a continuity with one another, transcending the conflicts of the past and building a solid bridge, one to the other, for the future.

We were abruptly brought back to reality when an orderly arrived with an oxygen tank, followed by another aide who placed Seymour on a stretcher and readied him for the elevator ride down to the surgery unit. We were allowed to accompany him and I held his hand throughout this last presurgery journey.

Just before his hospitalization, I used hypnosis to instruct Seymour to recognize my particular hand hold as a trigger to recall the meditation images and for entering his private world. He squeezed my hand, indicating that he had received the message. We gave him a hurried kiss good-bye and left him to his fate. The rest was up to him. We were all confident that he was up to the task and that we would see him again later that day.

Now started the waiting. It was 7 A.M. We wouldn't hear anything about the surgery's outcome for at least four hours, an eternity. I had already had a mild taste of hospital waiting rooms during Seymour's angiogram, and I didn't relish repeating that experience.

We went into the meditation room adjacent to the waiting room to say our prayers, my sons in their manner, I in mine. I suppose we all knew what was in the other's prayers and the sense of unity of spirit drew us together.

After breakfasting in the hospital cafeteria, we drove to a local park reserve. I suggested that we would be better off going for a walk in a park rather than sitting around in the hospital waiting room. Since we all love the outdoors, my suggestion was greeted warmly.

It was one of those perfect California mornings, the air clean and crisp, the coastal fog having just burned off. The sun was warm and gentle, more like a caress than a demand. The hills showed off the finery of their foliage, and the water sparkled with a gaiety of carefreeness. We were surrounded by nature's bounty and its serenity permeated every fiber of my being. It was hard to believe that I could be feeling sure and serene, while Seymour was undergoing the severe stress of surgery.

As the three of us walked and talked of times past, an openness developed among us. Our oldest son shared a confidence that he had never mentioned before. Our younger son, Zev, projected a sense of his manliness in his attention to my needs. They had matured into two fine young men who had all the characteristics required for mature living. They knew how to love, how to give, how to reach out and be with and for another person. My job as a mother was complete.

Was that the meaning of this episode in our lives—endings and beginnings? It seemed so. Our oldest son was moving to the east coast. Our younger son was expecting his second child. I had completed the task of mothering, and Seymour, yes Seymour, was at this very moment in the middle passage of his transformation. I looked at my watch. It was 10 A.M., time to head back. As my steps drew closer to our parked car, my heartbeat accelerated, not from the strain of the hike, but from the approach of the time of reckoning.

We arrived back at the hospital forty-five minutes later and I checked with the attending "candy striper" to see if there had been any word. There hadn't been. At this point, no news was good news.

I looked around at all the other anxious faces, each person engrossed in the silence of their own situation and feelings. We found a quiet corner for ourselves. Reading was impossible and watching television was unpleasant. I didn't want the external world to intrude on us. I was content to sit quietly and let my mind drift. Almost immediately it was drawn to images of Seymour in the surgery room. I sensed his aliveness and his pain.

About fifteen minutes had passed when I saw Dr. U., fully dressed in street clothing, and Dr. W., his assistant, still dressed in his surgery garb, approach us. They both had smiles on their faces. I jumped to my feet, my heart leaped into my throat. They uttered the first words, "All went well." Dr. U. suggested that we use the meditation room for privacy. We all sat around as he and his colleague described the surgery. It was a triple bypass, he told us, and then he described which blood vessels had been used as grafts. Apparently the condition of Seymour's coronary arteries was far worse than the angiogram had indicated. At best, he had probably had another few years of life in him and would have followed his father's path, death by age sixty-five.

I appreciated Dr. U.'s frankness and his willingness to talk to us in a calm and informative manner and to answer the children's questions. The surgery had gone without any complications. In fact, it had been accomplished quickly, in only three hours. In the days to come, the significance of the speed of the surgery would become more evident. The shorter the surgery, the shorter the time the body is stressed and the faster the recovery.

We were exuberant. I was tempted to give Dr. U. a kiss, but his manner told me that a hearty handshake was more appropriate. As we hurried to the phone, we saw Seymour being wheeled out of surgery to the intensive care unit. His face was gray, but not ashen as we had been told to expect. We called our daughter-in-law, who was waiting at home, and I could hear the relief in her voice and the strain that the waiting had placed on her. She must have been reliving her own father's surgery and death, and I wished I could console her. I knew that Seymour's survival would be the only meaningful consolation possible.

We were told that we could visit Seymour at 1:30 in the afternoon in the ICU. Suddenly I became aware of my ravenous hunger. We went to the hospital cafeteria and ate and talked somewhat hysterically. We no longer had to restrain our emotions. All we wanted now was a moment to be together with Seymour again.

We were allowed to visit Seymour in the ICU one at a time for fifteen minutes. I was the first to go in. Before I entered, I knew that I would be confronted with the full array of modern medical technology—tubes, telemetry machines, and so on. For someone like myself, not accustomed to the bionic world of modern medicine, this kind of setting can be overwhelming. And then to imagine Seymour in the midst of it all seemed unreal and horrible to contemplate. I had been warned that he would look quite ashen and would feel cold to the touch and that he would have multiple tubes and wires attached to him. In my imagination the scene had been frightening and devastating.

The reality was less horrific than I had imagined, and I felt relieved. Nonetheless, if there had been any doubt in my mind beforehand of the seriousness and severity of the operation, seeing Seymour with all those tubes coming out of his mouth, nose, neck, arms, and body convinced me that he had just gone through an ordeal I thought the human body could never tolerate. I had to force myself to focus on the *person* Seymour rather than on the *patient* Seymour.

He appeared to be reasonably comfortable. There were no discernible signs of pain or discomfort on his face. His breathing was assisted but regular. His body was cool but not cold, and his face was still gray. I was obviously searching for and finding signs to reassure me that indeed he was doing well. There were periodic tremors coursing through his body, as if his nervous system was attempting to awaken. The attending nurse was efficient, kind, and willing to answer my questions regarding his condition and the purpose and function of the various apparatuses.

I spoke to Seymour as I stroked his forehead and hands. He gave no sign of recognizing my presence or of knowing where he was or what had happened to him. The visit reassured me that he had transcended and would continue to transcend the trauma of the surgery. In the brief fifteen minutes I experienced a cacophony of emotions—joy, pain, sadness, hope, excitement, and confusion.

When I returned to the waiting room, I tried to prepare the boys for what they would see. I tried to project my feelings of joy and excitement, and keep the ones of sadness and pain to myself, at least for the moment.

After their visit, the three of us wearily returned home. Our conversation in the car continued on the note of intimacy and unity we had established earlier in the day. We all felt that we had experienced one of the most significant events in the history of our family, and we had all been deeply touched by it.

When we arrived home, we were greeted by our daughter-in-law who wanted to know about the events of the day in full detail. She too needed to feel included, as if she had been with us, and to participate in the sense of family unity. On our part, although weary and fatigued, we felt the need to retell the story in order to make it real and to etch the details in our minds.

Knowing that Seymour would probably not come out of his anesthetic stupor until the following morning, I decided that I would not return to the hospital for the evening visiting hour. However, after a short rest, I found myself wandering around the house feeling lost. I realized that I belonged at Seymour's side regardless of his state of awareness or my fatigue. At first it seemed silly to drive back to the hospital through one of the worst traffic corridors in our region, just to spend an additional few minutes with him. But logic was not the dominant variable ruling my actions. Emotions and needs rising from a deep internal well took over and I informed the children that I intended to return to the hospital that evening. They looked at me, at first incredulously. But in a moment they smiled, understanding my need and, in fact, they seemed pleased by my decision. I made it clear that I did not want them to accompany me. I wanted time alone with Seymour. Also, I needed an opportunity to be alone with my own thoughts and feelings.

After a hurried dinner, I left for the hospital and was immediately allowed into Seymour's room. He was now lying on his side, propped up by a triangular-shaped piece of foam. For some reason, whether it was because he was largely uncovered, or because of his position, or possibly because I was more focused in my attention, I was able to absorb more fully the reality of his condition. I noticed, for example, that his left leg, the one from which the vein had been removed, was bandaged from the top of his thigh to the toes.

I formed a mental picture of every tube protruding from his body and of the function of each one of them. I watched the video monitor and learned to read the continuous flow of information about his heart rate, pulse rate, and blood pressure. I was told that he had had two blood transfusions (procuring blood prior to surgery had been worth it), and that he had been given additional tranquilizers because he was beginning to gain consciousness prematurely. It was important to keep him out until his vital signs stabilized.

I had a need to know what everything meant, and, fortunately, the nurses answered all my questions. Most of all, I just wanted to be there with him, to hold his hand, stroke his forehead, and let him know that he was not alone. It appeared to me that his nervous system was responsive and that, on some level, he was aware of everything that had happened and was happening to him. I leaned over and gave him a gentle kiss and spoke softly to him. I reassured him that all had gone well and that he had done a great job. When I squeezed his hand, our private signal, he responded and returned the squeeze, ever so slightly. This was a magic moment. Despite the haze of anesthetics and tranquilizers I was able to connect and communicate with him. It was then that I understood why I had had to return to the hospital. It was for that hand squeeze, that signal.

A distinct pattern began to emerge. The rate of Seymour's recovery would remain one step ahead of our expectations and anxiety. For example, I believed that he would be incapable of responding, in any manner, to my physical presence only eight hours after surgery. But, in fact, he was able to do so. The following morning, twenty-four hours after surgery, when I saw him again, he was sitting up in bed, breathing on his own and able to speak. He had emerged from the anesthesia earlier that morning, at about 5 A.M., despite the nurses' efforts to keep him sedated the previous evening and night. He was clearly ready and desirous to return to the conscious world.

My excitement at witnessing his re-entry was matched only by his energetic response at finding himself alive and present. Despite the profusion of tubes coming out of his body, his energy was that of a healthy, mentally active, curious, socially present child. I say child because of the total lack of inhibitions or defensiveness on his part. It was as if he had been reborn.

I had to readjust my mental set and noticed a twinge of guilt as I did so. I had come to the hospital filled with apprehension about Seymour's condition and found that joy, excitement, and genuine happiness were more appropriate responses. I had underestimated Seymour and his capacity and willingness to recover quickly.

From the other rooms I heard hushed voices of concerned family members and occasional sounds of patients in pain. How could I be so joyous while others were far less fortunate? I repressed my ever-ready guilt so not to rob myself, my children, and, most important, Seymour of this exuberant moment of triumph.

Seymour clearly needed to talk. In his still husky, hoarse voice, he described, in a rush of words, his frustration earlier that morning, when he first returned to consciousness, at not being able to communicate with his nurse. He had had an insatiable need to know the time and day, how the surgery had gone, how many bypass grafts were done, how long had it taken, etc. He had needed to regain his bearings, identity, and command over himself. His nurse had not quite appreciated his intense curiosity and aliveness.

A second pattern emerged. The wished-for transformation Seymour and I had been working toward over the past several weeks was taking place before our eyes. Perhaps it was the after-effects of the surgery or of the sedation and anesthesia, but it seemed that the Seymour who greeted me that morning was the Seymour of his early childhood, not Seymour the recuperating patient. It was as if the years between age one and age sixty-two had been suddenly stripped away. I was thrilled with this wonderful "baby."

I stood back agog for I was suddenly struck by the similarity in personality between Seymour and our granddaughter. I realized that of course there would have to be a special bond between them. They recognized themselves in one another. I saw her playfulness and attracting sociability in him and his love for music and mindfulness in her.

We all knew that Seymour needed to have some form of contact with his granddaughter. Cheryl, our daughter-in-law, had the presence of mind to bring a photograph of her when they visited that afternoon and we clipped it to the back of the bed's footboard so that it would be in full view whenever Seymour sat up in bed.

And so the morning continued. Our fifteen-minute visit lasted about ninety minutes. Seymour's health and disposition hardly made us feel that we were visiting a person just twenty-four hours after surgery. If anything, it again felt festive. The cardiologist and surgeons arrived, examined him, gave their evaluation, wrote their orders, told us all was going well, and departed. All *was* proceeding well, it wasn't just my imagination.

While Seymour was napping, I left the hospital to find a men's store. I thought it would lift his spirits to have a snazzy new pair of pajamas so he could welcome his visitors looking like a distinguished gentleman rather than a sick hospital patient.

Thus, on a hot summer afternoon, while others were glued to their radios or television sets, watching the world apparently become unglued in the Persian Gulf, I prowled the nearby shopping mall, examining pajamas of various descriptions until I found the perfect pair. I was clearly creating my own reality.

When I returned to the hospital, I became aware of how tired I felt. The events of the past two days had wiped me out. It was unclear to me whether the fatigue I felt was the result of my body's knowing that it was safe now to let go or the fact that I had simply exhausted my resources. Whatever the case, I had to acknowledge my limitations and get some rest. There was still a long road ahead of us.

I recalled that one day after her husband's bypass surgery, a friend of ours slipped and broke her leg on the way to visit him in the hospital. Instead of being able to assist her husband, she ended up needing care herself and thus neither spouse could be helpful to the other. Given how I felt, I knew that I was vulnerable along similar lines. My judgment could easily become impaired and as a consequence I might get into an auto accident or in some other way injure myself just as our friend had. Also, out of sheer exhaustion I could possibly compromise my immune system and become ill or handicap myself in other ways. I had to keep telling myself that I was vulnerable and in danger. Awareness that one is in jeopardy is probably the best way of preventing harm or injury from happening.

At home that evening, the children had my dinner prepared and it was a wonderful feeling to be served and cared for. I gave them a full briefing on Seymour's condition and state of mind and they, in turn, gave me a report on their activities as well as on our granddaughter's latest antics. I longed for the time when everyone would be in bed and I could envelope myself in the peace and quiet of my own home. I needed time alone to gather my thoughts, process my feelings, re-establish a sense of internal well-being, and give my thanks. For the following few nights the midnight hours became my special time.

In the quiet of the night I contemplated how I felt about having survived the crisis of Seymour's surgery. I had put enormous mental and emotional preparation into the possibility of his not surviving, so I wondered whether or not, in some perverted way, I was disappointed. I was also aware of my penchant for the dramatic and, of course, death is much more dramatic than life. But when I dismissed the romantic, dramatic thoughts and contemplated the reality, his return to life filled me with an overwhelming sense of gratitude and joy.

I awoke the next day feeling refreshed and re-energized although I had had only five hours sleep. I looked forward to returning to the hospital and spending the day with Seymour. I wanted to be there when he was moved to the telemetry unit, his first major move after surgery. I arrived at about 10 A.M. to find him in excellent spirits and with fewer tubes emerging from his body. He was almost beginning to look human again.

He was interested in and responsive to my description of life at home, to which friends had called and inquired about him, etc., and he was just as enthusiastic about filling me in on the events of the past fifteen hours—how he had slept, how the noises of other patients in the unit had interfered with his sleeping, how cute the night nurse was, etc. He was preoccupied with bodily functions, his ability to breathe, drink, urinate, etc. For the ill person, these functions become the limits of their ego and the focus of their attention. Fortunately, Seymour was able to bring his good humor and optimism to bear on these preoccupations; otherwise it might have become boring and depressing.

We were waiting for the cardiologist and the surgeon to examine him and for the new room to be readied before the big move would occur. I noticed that Seymour took both opportunities to ask the doctors a lot of questions. His mind was still struggling with efforts to account for the time he was "out of it" and for "what happened." He was clearly uncomfortable with the missing spaces, and the attempt to string all the events together into a cohesive and meaningful whole would absorb him for many weeks to come.

The big moment arrived at 11:30 A.M. He not only was moved, but he did it under his own steam. He walked from the ICU, a nurse on one side and me on the other, each holding him under his arms. Seymour clutched a pillow against his chest and his oxygen tank rolled behind him as he slowly made his way to his new room, a good two hundred feet down the corridor. He moved step by step, smiling, greeting with a nod of his head anyone in the corridor—nurse, orderly, patient, or visitor. He was determined, and when he arrived at his goal he felt triumphant. It was a long march, and I could tell that he had to struggle. His energy was fading, but he was determined to make it on his own. This simple event became another challenge, another opportunity for him to experience success. By the time he reached his new room, he was thoroughly exhausted. I sensed that it had been too great a demand and said so to the nurse who accompanied us. She, a strong, stiff-lipped, do-or-die type, said, "Nonsense. It was good for him, sort of a test, a requirement for the transition."

He was now introduced to a new set of nurses who would be in charge of his welfare for the next three or so days. While in ICU the nurse-patient ratio was one to one. In the telemetry unit, the ratio was two to one, still quite intensive, but the patient no longer required nurses to hover and be immediately available.

Visiting hours were open all day in the telemetry unit, which meant I could remain with him or come and go as I wished. The room was large and airy, with a fine view of the bay and the San Francisco international airport. It was a comfortable private room and we made ourselves at home and settled in. Soon afterward, however, Seymour became cranky, almost like a sick two-year-old child. He pouted and whimpered as if he did not know what to do to feel physically better. (Psychologists call this reversion or backsliding to an earlier stage of development "regression.") The effects of the pain killers were obviously wearing off and he was experiencing greater discomfort than he had on the previous day. He was slowly becoming aware of the reality of what his body had gone through, and it was somewhat overwhelming.

In his psychologically regressed state, I had an opportunity to glimpse what Seymour's early childhood experience might have been like specifically as it related to his handling of bodily discomfort. Clearly, he had not been taught to self-soothe, nor did he seem to expect the adults around him to be helpful or understanding in providing comfort.

I recalled how his mother had responded to our own children when they were ill during their early years. She was concerned, but, at the same time she was quite helpless and unable to assist and comfort them. Instead, she went about fretting and wringing her hands. One wondered who required more assistance, her or the child. I assumed that when her own children had been ill, she had been equally discomforted and unable to be of much help. As I watched Seymour's apparent inability to come to grips with his pain, it was like seeing a young child reacting to a parent's inability to comfort and provide succor.

What a wonderful opportunity this state of regression offered for a re-education. First, I made sure that everything possible had been done for him physically. Then I began to teach him to respond to his body's needs in a more productive manner. He had learned to associate negative messages with such body signals as pain. I tried to reframe these signals with positive messages. For example, rather than identify the pain as a message of distress, I helped him redefine it as a signal that his body was healing. I also gave him suggestions as to how he might soothe himself—for example, by focusing on pleasant thoughts and future activities, or finding ways to rest and sleep. At one point, when his resistance was especially high, and he was convinced that he could not be comforted, I found myself scolding him as if he was indeed a child. He had been so successful in separating himself from his father during surgery, his task now, during the recuperative phase, as I saw it, was to separate himself psychologically from his mother.

When Elliot visited that afternoon, he picked up on the same theme without a cue from me. In a strong, almost stern voice, Elliot reminded Seymour that he was not an ill person and that he was in better shape internally than he had been before the surgery. He had to begin to think of himself as a healthy man, albeit for the time being in the process of regaining his energy and healing from the wounds of the surgery itself.

Seymour responded positively to these suggestions and began to calm down. I was right in feeling that too much may have been demanded of him when he was asked to walk from the ICU to his new room. It had drained what little energy he had and left him feeling less capable than the situation called for.

As I watched Seymour in the following few days it became more clear that the loss of physical ability was associated with a temporary loss of psychological ability. What I witnessed was a psychological regression to an earlier age of functioning, which itself was determined by the amount and degree of physical incapacity he was experiencing. It seemed that the process of recuperation mimicked the stages of psychological development one normally sees in childhood.

Because there was a replaying of developmental stages, there was also an opportunity for new learning to occur. I realized that I could help Seymour deal with old needs, fears, and attitudes in new and more adaptive ways. For example, the move to the telemetry unit made him aware of increased sensations of pain and discomfort and the extent and severity of the surgery. As a consequence, he became irritable, cranky, and whiney. By emphasizing and reminding him that there were alternative ways of responding, he was able to overcome the sense of trauma he apparently felt.

By late afternoon of the third day, Seymour's mood started to improve and we used this opportunity to take another walk, a much shorter one than previously, but nonetheless an opportunity for Seymour to experience his increasing ability. Walking is important not only for physiological recovery but also for psychological recovery. Just as patients are aware of their disability, they need to be aware of their ability. They need to feel that they are capable of mending. Seymour loved to walk down the corridor and show off his energy, willingness, and determination to anyone who would pay attention. The nurses were wonderful in giving him that recognition and encouragement, and I watched as he cheered up under the gaze of their approval. Again, how like a child at his best. Here regression was working for him; children thrive under the approving and delighted gaze of attending adults.

Before his surgery I feared that Seymour, as many in his position, might use the recuperative period as an opportunity to express his previously frustrated dependency needs. While I have little difficulty with those needs when they seem to be justified, I have little patience when they are exaggerated. I was, therefore, pleasantly surprised that he was not taking advantage of the situation. Quite the contrary. He showed a remarkable need for autonomy and self-sufficiency.

Thought of in terms of the recapitulation of developmental stages, Seymour was right on schedule. The issue of locomotion was being dealt with and autonomy and self-sufficiency were the next big issues to tackle. So far he was handling them with courage and pride.

On the fourth day Seymour continued to progress and while the family was visiting, one of Seymour's surgeons came by to examine him and to remove the last postoperative tube, a relatively large one inserted between his ribs for the purpose of draining fluids from his chest cavity. I did not want our grandchild to witness the scene, so I distracted her at the window, pointing out all the airplanes in the sky. Her father was standing next to Seymour, holding his hand, when the doctor yanked the tube out. The pain was excruciating, and I believe that without his son's support and the need to control himself because of his granddaughter's presence, he would have let out a howl that would have gotten the attention of everyone in the hospital and beyond.

He turned ashen and tried his best not to cry. The pain drained him of all his energy and he no longer could satisfactorily interact with us. His change of mood and disposition was notable. Children are sensitively perceptive of the changes in mood in the persons around them. Our granddaughter knew something happened and she had a look of concern on her face. I reassured her and she went off to explore the corridors and show off for the nurses. She seemed to recover much better than her father did. It was the first time that our son, Zev, had experienced first hand his father in pain and it had a profound effect on him.

Seymour needed time to rest and, despite a later visit from friends, his mood never quite recovered the rest of the day. We both wished that the medical procedure had been handled more adroitly and that he had been better prepared for it and/or given a local pain killer. I wondered if he experienced a sense of shame by being so exposed to his children, by being laid bare without preparation. The ego is so fragile at such points and the resources to deal adequately with unpleasant surprises are hardly available. While the surgeon meant well, I felt he might have been more sensitive to Seymour's emotional well-being.

When I arrived home that evening, my daughter-in-law took

me aside and informed me that Zev was feeling depressed. He felt that he had not been the help and support that his father needed. He was returning home in two days and he felt that his purpose and mission in coming had failed. In addition, he was feeling isolated from the rest of us. She appealed to me for help. I thanked her for the information, and suggested that after dinner we have a family talk. It had been a traumatic week and we all had a need for debriefing.

After dinner I gently moved the conversation to the emotional impact of the week and wondered how we all felt about our respective roles. I was pleased that Zev, who is usually reticent to talk about his feelings, allowed himself to be forthcoming. He felt that he hadn't given much to father. In light of the importance of his presence at his father's bedside that very afternoon, his revelation was startling. What could really be troubling him, I wondered.

I marveled at the contrast between the two brothers. The older one, Elliot, felt very involved and satisfied with his behavior. In fact, the experience with his father had helped him resolve many of the conflicts between the two of them and he felt connected to each and every one of us. He was feeling mature in the way he had handled himself. This week would become, in the weeks and months to follow, the genesis for much emotional growth for Elliot.

On the other hand, his brother had been burdened by a conflict that he had not yet resolved. Being an extremely caring and giving person, Zev felt the burden of giving his all both to his pregnant wife and child and to his family of origin. It was simply impossible to stretch his resources that far. He had to make some compromises, and he did. But his internal standard did not allow for compromises. He was, therefore, being hard on himself for not having lived up to his own standards. His depression stemmed from self-criticism and had less to do with our expectations than with his own. His sense of isolation arose from a sense of failure as compared to the rest of us who were feeling proud and satisfied with our efforts.

Airing his feelings in the context of a simultaneous affiliation with his new and old families allowed him to experience the unity between the two. The interests of both families were the same. Despite the fact that he had been married for five years, he was still feeling conflicted pulls of allegiance between his family of origin and his new one. He needed to feel an essential sense of belonging to both.

The closeness expressed that evening between us all went a long way in allowing Zev to form an image of both families as part of a larger all-encompassing unit. I think he was also moved by our concern for his welfare. Thus, despite his need to take care of others, he had an opportunity to receive some badly needed caring.

I went to sleep realizing that the surgery had offered not only Seymour but also every member of the family an opportunity to learn, relearn, and grow. An amazing healing was taking place in all of us. By the following morning, Zev's depressive feelings had lifted and he was able to devote his attention to his wife and child without feeling guilty that he was not attending to his parents' needs. In the hospital that day, Dr. U., Seymour's primary surgeon, came to visit. He examined Seymour and was pleased with his progress. Then he sat back and embarked on what appeared to be the main purpose of his visit—encouraging Seymour to exert his energy, to think of himself as a healthy man, and to keep up his daily walks as much as possible. He suggested, for example, that when Seymour went back home, he not spend his days in bed, but rather that he dress, eat his meals at a table, and get out of the house as often as possible. In other words, he described a routine that included all the symbols of normality and health rather than of illness and debilitation. These were just the words that Seymour needed and wanted to hear because they corresponded perfectly with his own will and determination and were the perfect antidote to the concerns about the ubiquitous depression everyone predicted would follow bypass surgery. The upbeat tone of his voice was not an act. The man truly believed that one's mental stance had an effect on one's physical recovery.

I told Dr. U. about our sons and their struggles, witnessing their father's crisis. His response was typical of him. He thought it was important that they not be shielded from the experience because it provided them with an inoculation of reality that would help them deal with the fact that they might have inherited a genetic predisposition toward atherosclerosis. They needed to face that possibility, and the time was *now* for them to start taking matters into their own hands. He didn't mince words. He didn't protect. He stated reality clearly, but didn't make a tragedy out of it. He stood for the principle of using knowledge to control fate.

I watched Seymour absorb every word Dr. U. uttered. His presentation of the prospects for the immediate and distant future were both encouraging and realistic. In essence, he told Seymour that he could have the future he wished, but that it would take effort and willingness on his part. That type of encouragement was particularly useful since Dr. U. spoke with authority and knowledge.

The effect of Dr. U.'s visit on Seymour's mood was visible. He even started to get some color back in his face. That afternoon Seymour was moved again, this time back to the eighth floor, the floor on which he had started his journey the previous Monday. He was recognized and greeted by the floor nurses like a conquering hero returning from the wars. This move was much less disturbing for him because it was back to a familiar space and because his ego was able to arouse the necessary skills to cope with the change. The move also had an important symbolic value. It indicated that he no longer required extra special care and that it was time to prepare for the return home. The fact that the room was less pleasantly appointed than the previous one increased his motivation to return home.

The speed with which Seymour recovered was greater than either one of us had been prepared for. It appeared that he was likely to be discharged on Monday, six days after the surgery. I found myself surprised at my mixed feelings. Surely I was pleased with his visibly increasing strength, normal facial coloration, and more normal sociability. And surely having him home would mean he was entering another phase of his recovery. Yet, I found myself fretting about that return.

During a quiet time in the afternoon, I went out for a long walk to sort out my feelings and clarify my thoughts. I had begun to fall into a routine—days in the hospital, nights alone at home. In a strange way it felt safe. I knew that Seymour was being well taken care of. When I left him each day I could focus my attention on my own needs and thoughts. Once I had him home, it felt like I would need to take over all the functions of the nurses and doctors. I would have to perform not only to satisfy my own demanding standards, but also because Seymour would be dependent on the quality of my care. I wasn't sure what that meant in actual terms, nor was I sure I could perform all the required tasks adequately. The responsibility weighed heavily on me. I wished I had been given guidelines, instruction, or training— something—to better prepare me for the forthcoming challenges. I couldn't share these concerns with Seymour. It was important, or so I thought, that he have every confidence in my ability to care for him fully.

My anticipatory anxiety was beneficial in this case. It was only Saturday, I reminded myself. I still had two days in which to prepare. I clearly needed information about what to expect, and how to respond to Seymour's special needs. I needed to be present when his doctors came around so that I could talk to them and obtain answers to my questions.

As I continued my walk and inner dialogue I became aware of how unreal and disconnected I felt. I watched people gardening, driving, performing simple, normal activities, but I felt completely apart from their reality. I felt invisible or like an alien creature. I seemed numb. I couldn't feel the sensation of walking, or the sun on me, or the air moving around me—whether out of anxiety, fatigue, or disbelief, I wasn't sure. Perhaps because of all three. I asked myself what I was doing in this town, walking these streets alone on a summer Saturday afternoon.

The events of the past week had not yet been incorporated into my reality. I had lived them, but they had not yet become a part of me. Things had moved so swiftly that before I could adapt to one phase of the surgery and recovery, it was over and another phase had begun. My capacity for adaptation was being stretched to the limit.

I felt the urge to return to the hospital and to be with Seymour as if a leash was tugging at me, and I became aware that if I focused on him, I could reduce the effect of the environment. I returned to his room and found him asleep. I felt secure again. My place was at his side, because that was where I needed to be to feel my own reality.

Early Sunday morning, Zev and his family left for home in the midwest. More change. They were gone and in a few days our other son would also leave for the east coast. My sadness at their departure brought to mind our constant refrain, "Its just you and me, kid." I had come closer than ever before to experiencing the possibility of losing the "you" in that refrain. And then it would have been, "It's just me." I was sad, but not empty.

Going home increased in reality as we discussed the details of his discharge, such as which items of clothing he wanted to wear and what foods he wanted me to prepare for him. Things became even more concrete when I took home some of the flowers friends had brought, the get-well cards, and some extraneous items in order to lessen the burden the following day. Homecoming was going to be the final and most welcomed change.

Monday morning, I tried to arrive at the hospital as early as I could, but, unfortunately, was delayed in traffic. I say unfortunately because I missed his doctor's visit and I had promised myself that I would be there. When I arrived, Seymour was already up and about, restlessly waiting for me. I helped him put on his street clothes and watched the delight on his face. He was no longer a patient. His status had instantly changed.

The supervisory nurse arrived to say good-bye and to give us both last-minute instructions and encouraging words. We were ready to leave. A volunteer arrived and brought Seymour down in a wheelchair to the front of the hospital while I brought the car around. It had been a trying but triumphant week.

Once in the car, Seymour became overwhelmed with emotion. Tears rolled down his face as he looked around him. The world looked exactly the same as it had a week before, but from his perspective it was all different. On the almost hour-long drive home, he pointed out the many familiar sights and sounds we passed as if it was the first time he was really seeing them.

While Dr. U. claimed that his life hadn't really changed, in fact it had. Seymour's bypass surgery was not an isolated event that could be compartmentalized without touching other aspects of his and our lives. Its meaning had to be faced and incorporated, and that task as well as others awaited him as he began the next phase of his recovery.

FIVE

· · · · · · · · · · ·

LIFE AFTER SURGERY

Even after you leave the hospital following surgery, you are not finished with the medical system. There will generally be several more visits to the surgeon's office, perhaps to take stitches out and certainly to check on your progress in healing. In addition, decisions about your life have to be made.

Most patients recover from the surgery without any major postsurgical complications. Each day brings increasing strength and the ability to do the things you used to do in the past. However, a new set of psychological issues arises after you leave the hospital, and how they are dealt with may determine the quality of your life in the weeks, months, and years ahead.

RETURNING HOME

Leaving the hospital after the surgery often gives you the sense that you are seeing the world afresh, as if for the first time. Your time sense, altered by the medications and drugs you received, may not have returned, and you may feel out of touch with the world for a long period of time. Reentry often brings with it a sense of enormous joy and renewal, which, in turn, may bring tears to your eyes and a sense of overwhelming emotion. One man described his homecoming as follows:

> I entered my home and slowly walked from room to room reacquainting myself with each space, lightly touching each piece of furniture, letting my fingers comb through the potted ferns, looking at the pictures on the various walls, pausing to look at the vista visible through our living room sliding door, the Golden Gate Bridge and the city of San Francisco off in the distance. The warmth of the day mingled with the delightful kitchen aromas of foods recently prepared, some of my favorites. . . .

Many bypass graduates report that simple things—a flower, a familiar scent, a scrap of music, a child at play, watching a football game on television—may bring on a flood of feelings. To the extent that you are accustomed to experiencing and expressing these "soft" feelings, you will either find satisfaction and release or distress and anxiety as you realize that your attempts to control tears and feelings do not work.

Unfortunately some health professionals have tended to misinterpret this easy emotionality following bypass surgery to mean that the patient is either depressed or becoming depressed. On the whole, this may be a misreading of the situation. The patient has been opened emotionally, and as a result, his or her emotions are closer to the surface—more accessible. Opening the heart appears to remove the psychological defenses we usually use to bury our emotions. Thus, feelings of emotional connection to things, significant others, and oneself are readily available to the postsurgical patient. This is just the opposite of what happens in a depression, when the person's self-esteem has been battered and one's mood is dominated by feelings of helplessness and hopelessness.

Mental health professionals sometimes promote the idea that depression is almost inevitable after bypass surgery. Much of the literature about heart bypass fails to make a distinction between depression, which often has a paralyzing effect and harms a person's self-esteem, and sadness, which is not debilitating and leaves a person's self-esteem intact. Sadness and increased emotionality are normal responses to the changes we perceive in our life and relationships as a result of heart disease or bypass surgery. To mislabel such responses as depression may be a disservice to patients.

One of the things I recall from the presurgical and immediate postsurgical period was the repeated warnings I received about the depression bypass patients invariably suffer afterwards. Many nurses, doctors, and technicians said something to the effect, "Don't be surprised if you get depressed. Everyone who has a bypass operation becomes depressed." The recovering patient tends to hear that warning over and over again and after a while it takes on a self-fulfilling quality.

The overemphasis on predicting depression may in itself promote depression. I believe that what professionals may be trying to communicate is that the patient's energy might not be as available as it had been in the past. After bypass surgery many persons report that they tended to "fade" earlier in the day and to become fatigued more frequently than they had before the surgery. These periods of low energy are not usually accompanied by the hallmarks of clinical depression—dysphoric mood, feelings of worthlessness, low self-esteem, and suicidal thoughts. When one's energy wanes, it could lead to depressive feelings, but they are not as invariable as some health professionals make them out to be.

By framing the postsurgical psychological reactions in negative terms, professionals may unwittingly contribute to the incidence of depression seen following bypass surgery. Professionals need to provide a more positive approach, one that gives patients a basis for building on successes as they heal and return to health. The expected waxing and waning of a person's energy following the surgery should be normalized as essential to the process of recovery, rather than being presented as a precursor of psychological difficulty. Some of the good advice physicians might give patients is, "No matter how you feel, get dressed each day, shave (put on make up), and prepare yourself for activity. Do not become a couch potato. Avoid television watching. If you are tired, rest up, take a nap. Plan an activity for each day. Walk as much as you can, several times a day. Think about health. Give yourself messages: 'Heal,' 'Be healthy.' "

Obviously, should a person actually become depressed, one's physician should be notified immediately. Among the major telltale signs of depression to look for are thoughts about suicide or a diminished desire to live, a loss of interest or pleasure in one's usual activities, a general state of apathy, feelings of worthlessness and unusual negative thoughts about oneself, sleep disturbances such as persistent insomnia, and a persistent "down" mood.

It would also be important for professionals to normalize the emotional lability many patients experience for several weeks, sometimes months, after surgery. My wife and I went out to dinner with another couple about two months after my surgery, and at the end of the meal, as we reached for our respective credit cards to pay the bill, my friend said, "No, no, this is our treat to celebrate your successful surgery and recovery." I felt overwhelmed by their gesture of affection, and seated at the table in this public place, I broke into tears, sobbing for what felt like several minutes. One can sometimes feel so good about being alive, so valued by others, so much in touch with the essence of life that the only reasonable response is to let the tears of triumph and joy flow unrestrained.

If you are not accustomed to emotional release in this manner, it might be important to understand that waves of inner emotional warmth often become released when the heart is touched, literally or emotionally. Looking at a flower, a bird, a sunset, a remembered thought or song, a scene on television, a phrase in a book, a smile, a lift of the head, any one of these things may be sufficient to bring tears and release waves of warmth. When this occurs, an aspect of the self, perhaps long suppressed, is being expressed like a reminder of the human capacities available to most of us. Bypass surgery appears to open the person up on more than a physical level. There is a psychological opening as well that gives you an opportunity to recognize aspects of yourself that over time have become unfamiliar and alien. This recognition and acceptance of these aspects of yourself can bring about or promote important changes in your life.

Several months after my own surgery, I came across a book that suggested that many patients who have bypass surgery tend to become depressed on the fifth postsurgical day, implying that the depression is due to the surgery. However, this depression corresponds to the time when patients are moved to quarters other than the ICU or telemetry units. Thus, one has to wonder what role this move and other situational factors—such as having a chest drainage tube removed or seeing visitors—have in inducing the mood changes. To my knowledge, no one has carried out research on these important issues. Thus, a mythology, which may have little or no scientific basis, has begun to build around the emotional effects of bypass surgery.

As a postsurgical patient, you ought to expect that no two days will be alike in terms of how energetic you might feel. Generally patients reported that they had more energy in the mornings and that when their energy waned, it did so suddenly. Several persons described it thus: "It's as if someone pulled the plug." This sudden depletion may be accompanied by chills, enormous fatigue, and an urge to lie down and go to sleep. This too is a normal response to what the person has experienced and is part of the healing process. Individuals who have had a heart attack or perioperative complications may have a greater need for such periods of physical and emotional recharging. The need to rest when the body tells you it's time to do so should be respected.

The most difficult task during the first few days after coming back home may be to learn how to get out of bed on your own. Because of the surgical chest wound and the fact that the breastbone, wired during surgery, requires maximum immobilization, the muscles one generally uses to move from a lying to a sitting position cannot be called totally into action to accomplish this simple task. This means that it may be difficult to sit up unassisted. This also means that you may need assistance in order to go to the bathroom in the middle of the night or during the day. Most persons seem to figure out within a week a way of turning on the side, dropping their legs off the bed so as to give momentum to pivot to a sitting position. In my case, this was a major step toward autonomy that freed the two of us. It allowed my wife to return to work knowing that I was ready to take over some of my caretaking.

DEVELOPING A ROUTINE

Perhaps when you were discharged from the hospital you were given instructions about the breathing, stretching, and other exercises you might do back home (if not ask your physician for advice). These exercises will contribute to your healing, and thus you should include them in your daily routine.

It is also strongly advisable to develop a daily routine that includes rising early rather than sleeping late, showering or bathing, shaving, and so on. Perhaps after breakfast and a short rest, go out for a walk. At first you will need a companion, but within a short period of time you may be able to manage a walk on your own. Try to plan two or three such short walks each day, weather permitting, unless your physician advises you otherwise.

At the beginning a walk may consist of a slow spin to the corner and back. However, usually before the first week is over, you may find that you want to attempt a greater challenge such as a gradual incline. You may want to measure your progress by the number of houses or other landmarks you pass on your walk. This gives you concrete evidence of your growing recovery.

Because your leg may still be edematous (swollen with fluid), you may need to keep it raised on pillows when in bed. When seated, keep it up on a pillow placed on the back of a chair or table so that it is higher than your heart. This allows the fluid in the leg to drain. Walking also helps to keep the leg swelling down and promotes the development of collateral circulation to compensate for the vein that was removed in the surgery.

If you have prepared yourself for bypass surgery by using meditation or similar techniques, the return home offers further opportunity to use such procedures for the purposes of promoting healing and other important tasks. When you require rest or after having taken a rest may be an excellent time to meditate or to visualize the healing process. Several times a day find time to close your eyes in a quiet place and to focus your attention on one or more of the following:

1. Your chest and breast bone: Visualize how the cells in this area are working together actively to mend the surgical wound. Provide encouragement to them. Tell them to heal.
2. Your leg: Repeat the messages described above.
3. Your body: Tell it how much you appreciate it and how courageous it was. Tell it that you know how much it hurts and that soon it will be well and strong again.
4. Your new "arteries": Visualize them. See how open and strong they are. Ask them what they need from you. Tell them how you will care for them.
5. Your heart: Thank it for beating and returning you to life. Tell it how you plan to care for it and keep it healthy. Listen to the feelings it has to tell you about.

MEMORY AND CONCENTRATION PROBLEMS

Several postsurgical patients told me that soon after they returned home from the hospital, they began to ask their significant others for help in reconstructing the sequence of events immediately before and after the surgery, when they were still sedated. I recall doing the same thing with Hilda. It seemed so strange to me, almost amusing, when I was told that I had said such and such to so-and-so and I could recollect nothing about it. What was even stranger was that I found I could not keep the information she gave me straight in my mind. So we went through several rounds of the following: "Hon, I know you told me how it went, but I wonder if you wouldn't mind going through it again for me. I just can't seem to comprehend it. I woke up out of the anesthesia, when? When did they remove the endotracheal tube?"

I began to wonder if my memory had been impaired by the surgery or by the anesthetics I had been given. I had read that other individuals who had bypass surgery had memory problems later on, although I have never found corroborating evidence to this effect. Nonetheless, the anesthesia experience seems to sensitize the person to indications of memory dysfunction, and it becomes easy to attribute small lapses of memory to the surgery or the anesthesia used in the surgery rather than to other plausible factors. It needs to be remembered that as we age normally, memory seems not to be as sharp as it once was. It is almost impossible to differentiate the slips of memory due to aging from those possibly due to the surgery or the anesthetics. In one or two instances, spouses of bypass patients told me that their respective mates had episodes of confusion while still in the hospital, but this was a transient phenomenon.

Several weeks after I came home, a friend telephoned to inquire how I was doing, and in the course of conversation she mentioned that it would be nice to get together for dinner sometime. Several weeks later I suddenly recalled that our friend had phoned, and I panicked. I was convinced that she had invited us for dinner, that I had neglected to mention it to Hilda, and that the date had already passed. I was certain that we had missed the dinner, inconvenienced our friends, and embarrassed ourselves. Hilda stayed cool and merely said, "Call her up and straighten it out." When I did, our friend was completely understanding. "No. No definite date had been set for the dinner. But since you're calling, let's set a date now."

All's well that ends well. Nonetheless, it is evident how one's self-confidence might be shaken by a trivial event of that kind. In my case, I developed the habit of being extraconscientious about writing things down, so as to avoid such potential "disasters."

Some postsurgical patients report that their ability to concentrate seems affected by the surgery, particularly when they attempt to do work-related activities or read books. This too appears to be a transient phenomenon. Several individuals I spoke to read short newspaper articles, "lightweight" novels, and/or listened to books on audiotape after they came home from the hospital. Others listened to music. Many watched too much television or rented videotapes of movies. Reading is an exceptional way of keeping your mind actively occupied, and some of the persons I talked to used reading as a way of monitoring their postsurgical progress. They found that their ability to concentrate and to absorb what they read tended to increase each day, leaving them feeling that they were healing and returning to normality. This would have an obvious positive effect on their overall mood.

SEX AND THE BYPASS GRADUATE

One of the questions frequently posed to physicians by bypass graduates is, "When can I start having sex again?" Often the answer is, "As soon as you're ready." Feeling ready, however, may be a complex matter—and so is having sex. For some, sexual activity may consist of hugging, kissing, and gentle touching or caressing, generally, but not necessarily, involving the genitals. For others, sex may consist of Olympic acrobatics. After a heart attack or bypass surgery you may experience a lack of confidence in your sexual abilities, and you may be concerned about when and if you can return to pre-illness or presurgical levels of sex. Available guidelines put out by the American Heart Association (AHA) and by others suggest that over 80 percent of persons who had a heart attack resume sexual activities between four and six weeks after the heart attack (if in doubt, check with your physician). Also, about 75 percent of individuals who have had bypass surgery appear to resume having sex with the same frequency (and using same sexual positions) as they did before the surgery.

Sexual activity for persons who have had bypass surgery may be influenced by three factors. First, soon after the surgery there may be discomfort in the chest, arms, and other parts of the body due to the surgery, and this discomfort may limit the kinds of positions they can take. The discomfort may also promote concerns about the heart itself and remind partners that there was a "problem" with this organ.

Second, the heart and its ability to "hold out" during sex is a frequent concern among sex partners. Heart rate and blood pressure both increase during sex and generally reach a high point during orgasm. The heart rate may increase from 90 to 145 beats per minute during orgasm, with an average peak of about 115 beats per minute. Generally the revascularized heart that results after bypass surgery can handle this demand with ease since this level is maintained only for about 15–20 seconds and then tends to decline rapidly to resting levels. If you experience angina symptoms, you should obviously slow down, reduce your exertions, rest, and take the medicines your physician has prescribed. Also, let your physician know about it.

Third, one of the things that limits sexuality and intimacy between couples is their perceptions of their bodies. If we feel unattractive, we do not generally put out "come hither" messages. On the contrary. We often reject or do not respond to sexual overtures when, inwardly, we feel repulsive. This may occur between mates after bypass surgery because the patient has scars from the surgery and may feel he or she is repugnant to the mate. Initially mates may be repelled, but those feelings often tend to wane. More commonly, patients feel sensitive about being touched in the chest area and evade such contact as if they were protecting themselves from further injury. How spouses can deal with this situation is discussed in the next chapter.

UNDERSTANDING FRIENDS AND RELATIVES

How friends and relatives respond during the postoperative period requires comment. Many patients report that once they informed their friends and relatives they were going to have surgery, the phone literally jumped off the hook. Everyone seemed to call to find out what was going on, to express their concern and support, and to wish the person well. Frequently they tell the spouse that if there is anything they can do to help, to please call on them. The sheer number of calls can be overwhelming. Although the desire to express concern and to help is frequently genuine and sincere, other factors are often operating. First, when a peer's life and health are threatened, we become fearful about our own health. We feel personally vulnerable. If it can happen to him or her, it can also happen to me.

Second, when a friend or relative is in crisis, we sense a loss of control over our universe. Control is restored either through active support of the other or through actively moving to safer ground and distancing oneself from the sick person. Support is often welcomed and appreciated; however, the distancing that may occur can be puzzling and disappointing to the bypass patient. Sometimes friends respond to the patient as if they needed to protect themselves. It is almost as if bypass surgery were a communicable disease and by keeping their distance they are protecting their own health.

Third, we all have a desire to help, reach out, show support. For some, these activities come easily. But for others, even if the desire is present, the expression of support makes them uncomfortable or uneasy. The latter may feel unsure or ineffectual in their attempts or vulnerable that their supportive efforts might be seen as inadequate. Some are concerned about being too intrusive. Thus, some friends remain close to the patient throughout the entire surgical and postsurgical period. They call, they visit, they take you out for walks, they bring food. In short, they are thoughtful and helpful. On the other extreme, there are friends who never call, never send a card, never make their concern known, even though they know that you have had surgery. Usually it is not that they are unconcerned or uncaring. No. It is simply that they do not know how to show or express their feelings. Some feel so inept in this regard that all they can do is keep their distance. Under different circumstances, when the another's health is not involved, these same friends may behave in a socially appropriate manner.

In the postsurgical period, the most touching and helpful acts of friends often consist in bringing food over or simply coming to visit the patient and his or her significant other. One of our neighbors brought over an entire cooked (zero cholesterol and low fat) meal, on platters, with silverware, served it, and cleaned and washed up afterwards. This was much appreciated.

Many people think that after surgery the patient wants to be left alone. This is not the experience of many postsurgical persons. Many value and enjoy the attention that comes with visits from friends, no matter how short the visit. Perhaps it is the vulnerability and/or the need for self-centeredness during the immediate postsurgical period, but many individuals appear to thrive on the attention of family and friends when the latter give of themselves and put themselves out for the postsurgical individual. However, when patients felt that friends and relatives were taking or that they had to reassure them that they were doing fine, they saw the experience as emotionally empty and draining.

Some patients seem to expect that visitors will drain them. Perhaps because they feel personal shame and embarrassment about the surgery, they tend to shun or set up obstacles to visits by friends. Such individuals or couples are, in my experience, prone to depressive reactions and should be monitored closely by the medical community. Turning away from others and social isolation are signs of depression.

The fact that no two people will respond in the same way to new circumstances was brought home to me following my own surgery. About three weeks after the surgery, we received a call from some friends who asked us whether or not it would be possible for us to get out and join them for dinner. They planned the dinner to take place early enough so that my energy would not be depleted. Also, it was made explicit that as soon as my energy began to wane, I would be expected to leave. I felt that my friends were taking my needs into consideration and that accommodations were being made to help me return to the social scene, to see and to be with my friends. So we ventured it, and I even made it through the main course before I felt my energy start to give out. We went home immediately, and I had the sense of good feelings all around. I felt cared for and emotionally nourished. From my point of view it felt like a triumph.

In contrast, a week later, we were invited to a dinner at which I was treated as if all was normal. At this friend's home a dinner invitation generally means a set protocol, including obligatory canapés accompanied and followed by banter and discussions of political, philosophical, and intellectual matters. In normal circumstances this is stimulating and provides intellectual sustenance. However, on this particular occasion, by the time the food was brought out my energy was completely depleted, and I was feeling chilled. I tried my best to put on a brave face and to hang in there so as not to hurt my hosts' feelings. I went through the motions of being physically present, but psychologically I was withdrawn and left before the dinner was over, feeling battered.

One of most profound lessons many people learn following major surgery is that the reactions of others have more to do with their own limitations than with their feelings of friendship and affection. In order to cope with possible disappointment about the reactions of friends, try to think of times when the tables were turned—when friends needed you to extend yourself, to put yourself out for them. How many of us have been models of virtue? We sometimes let our friends down because of our own discomfort and thoughtlessness, not out of lack of feeling for them. If you are able to let go of judgmental feelings and become more accepting and tolerant of others' limitations, you will have learned something valuable indeed.

Major life events such as bypass surgery often affect relationships with others, particularly friends. It is not unusual for friendship patterns to change, sometimes dramatically, following a major life stress. The person or persons most affected by the stress often feel disappointed by the reactions of others. These reactions are frequently experienced as being inadequate, inappropriate, insensitive, ill-timed, too little, too late. Following surgery, you are likely to feel very vulnerable and overly sensitive to others' awkwardnesses, insensitivities, and bumbling attempts to convey caring and thoughtfulness. Also, you will no doubt feel needy, perhaps as part of your effort to undo the injury you have suffered by the surgery, and no amount of attention and caring of friends can undo this wound. This promotes a sense of disappointment in others, which, if not checked, can lead to the abandonment of friends and friendships, even long-standing ones.

The rejection of friends is often an acting out of the inner experience of having felt abandonned by others in one's own hour of need. This may lead to a real isolation from others, which may then be interpreted as further evidence that one has been abandoned. Behavior that leads you to isolate yourself from others and feelings of disappointment at friends' inept responses need to be carefully examined—with enormous tolerance for yourself and your friends. You may need to make peace with the fact that friends are not perfect and that they cannot always come through for you, especially to fill the huge needs created by your vulnerability at this particular time. Friends, regardless of their limitations and imperfections, are valuable assets—assets to be treasured rather than cast away.

DEVELOPING LIFE GOALS AFTER SURGERY

The goal of life after a bypass ought to be the maintenance, for as long as possible, of the gains achieved by surgery. For most individuals, simple changes in diet, lifestyle alterations, increased exercise, weight reduction, and stress reduction may be all that is needed to maintain health. For others, especially individuals with an inherited predisposition to heart disease, medications may also be needed.

Recently, Dr. Dean Ornish and his colleagues at the University of California School of Medicine at San Francisco have suggested that lifestyle changes, including a low-fat, vegetarian diet, stopping smoking, moderate exercise, and stress management through a combination of stretching exercises, breathing techniques, meditation, Progressive Relaxation, and imagery, may promote a reversal of coronary atherosclerosis without the use of cholesterol-lowering medications.

In a study published in the British journal *Lancet,* Ornish and his co-workers assigned persons with documented CAD to either an experimental or control group. The experimental group was placed on a low-fat, vegetarian diet that included fruits, vegetables, grains, legumes, and soybean products. All meat, poultry, and fish were eliminated. The only animal products allowed in the diet were egg whites and one cup per day of nonfat milk or yogurt. The daily cholesterol intake was restricted to about 5 mg or less, and the diet contained about 10 percent of its calories as fat. Caffeine was entirely eliminated from the diet. The twenty-two experimental subjects were also asked to exercise for no less than three hours per week and to spend at least an hour each day in carrying out the stress management techniques. In addition, these individuals participated in twice-weekly group discussions designed to provide social support and to help them adhere to the program. At these group meetings, each of which lasted four hours, the members discussed strategies for maintaining the lifestyle changes; they were taught communication skills and were encouraged to express their feelings about interpersonal relations at work and at home.

The nineteen persons in the control group were not asked to make any lifestyle changes, although they were free to do so if they chose. However, presumably they were encouraged by their physicians to effect changes in their diets, exercise routines, and stress management. In contrast to the experimental group, the control individuals did not have the benefit of group support to adhere to whatever lifestyle changes they made.

After one year, the researchers compared the two groups on

multiple measures and found that the people in the experimental group reported a 91 percent reduction in the frequency of angina symptoms, whereas those in the control group reported a 165 percent increase in such symptoms. The former also had a 42 percent reduction in the duration of their angina episodes and a 28 percent reduction in the severity of angina. The persons in the control group, on the other hand, reported increases of 95 percent in the duration of and 39 percent in the severity of angina episodes.

When the angiogram results were examined after one year in the study, it was found that the average degree of occlusion of the coronary arteries of the persons in the experimental group decreased from 40.0 percent to 37.8 percent, whereas among the individuals in the control group it increased from 42.7 percent to 46.1 percent. When only the more severe occlusions were analyzed, the experimental group showed a decrease from 61.1 percent to 55.8 percent, whereas the control group showed an increase from 61.7 percent to 64.4 percent.

Overall, 82 percent of the individuals in the experimental group showed a regression in the degree of coronary artery occlusion, whereas only 42 percent of the control group showed such regression and 53 percent showed a progression of coronary atherosclerosis.

This research is difficult to assess because the sample size was small and multiple variables were studied simultaneously. For example, it is impossible to know what role the group support—which, because of the way the study was structured, differentiated the two groups—had on the overall results irrespective of the exercise and stress management procedures. Also, support groups often engender a group "mind-set," a kind of peer pressure, which might have promoted the underreporting of angina symptoms. In addition, the degree of regression of coronary artery occlusion among the experimental subjects was not over-whelmingly large, and almost half of the persons in the control group, who did not share the regimen of the experimental sub-jects, also showed some regression.

Many clinicians and researchers in the field are not yet con-vinced by Ornish's research and would like to see an indepen-dent replication of his studies. Nonetheless, whether or not the findings withstand the test of time, Ornish has succeeded in bringing the problem of CAD and its relationship to lifestyle activities to a wide audience—his books have become bestsell-ers—and his argument that lifestyle changes may be able to halt or reverse coronary atherosclerosis without the use of drugs has broad appeal. His research suggests that the persons who made the greatest changes in lifestyle tended to show the greatest im-provement in reducing their atherosclerosis. For persons who have had bypass surgery, Ornish's findings suggest that if they are willing to adopt health-promoting regimens—eating right, ex-ercising, managing stress more effectively—they may be able to maintain their cardiac well-being for longer periods of time than persons who return to their old, familiar habits.

Almost all professionals believe that Ornish's recommenda-tions about diet, exercise, reduction of stresses in one's life, prac-tice of mind-body techniques, and social support, all have enor-mous merit. However, not all professionals feel that everyone has the self-discipline, capacity, or desire to adhere to the de-manding diet and lifestyle regimen he advocates. Nonetheless, there are some common sense things bypass graduates should do to maintain their cardiac health that come close to Ornish's rec-ommendations, and these will be discussed below. For example, if you have not already done so, stop smoking. Smoking signifi-cantly increases your risks for coronary artery disease and cancer. If you cannot stop smoking on your own, join a support group, such as Smokers Anonymous, devoted to helping you quit. Ask your doctor for help or contact the American Cancer Society or the American Lung Association for information and assistance. If you try to quit smoking on your own, remember to develop rewarding, health-promoting behaviors to substitute for ones you are abandoning.

EATING RIGHT

Whether or not you adopt the specific diet advocated by Ornish, as a bypass graduate you will need to make major changes regarding food. The aim of dietary changes is to help lower blood cholesterol levels since high levels of this substance are a major risk factor contributing to CAD (see Chapter 1). Medications may also be used for this purpose. In several studies in which patients were randomly assigned to experimental and control groups, it has recently been shown that regression (reversal) of atherosclerosis in coronary arteries and in bypass grafts can be achieved through the use of cholesterol-lowering medications. Medications, however, may have their risks. For example, some individuals on a high niacin regimen may show (reversible) liver function abnormalities. Psychological approaches, such as meditation, may, for some individuals, bring results comparable to those achieved by medications, without the additional risks. For individuals with a genetic predisposition to high cholesterol levels, a combination of diet, medication, and psychological approaches may be necessary.

To maintain your cardiac health, you will need to develop new eating habits that emphasize only low-fat, low-cholesterol foods. When you shop, read the food labels. Labels are now required to give you important information about the cholesterol and fat content of the food you buy. If the fat content is not broken down into monounsaturated/polyunsaturated and saturated fats, assume that the fat is saturated, that is, not healthy. Saturated fat contributes to high cholesterol levels, which, in turn, promote the clogging of your arteries. The American Heart Association suggests that you avoid foods high in saturated fats such as butter, cream, red meats, whole milk, cheese, chocolate, and coconut and restrict foods high in cholesterol such as egg yolks, liver, and other organ meats. If you want to keep your arteries unclogged, err on the conservative side—avoid foods containing cholesterol or saturated fats.

Ideally, on a daily basis, no more than 10 percent of your caloric intake should come from monosaturated or polyunsaturated fats. You can determine how close you come to this ideal by calculating the caloric content of your daily meals—many cookbooks have tables showing the nutritional content of various foods—and multiplying the total calories by 0.1. For example, if your total caloric intake per day is about 2000 calories, then no more than 200 calories should come from fat. Since each gram of fat provides about nine calories, your daily fat intake should not exceed 22 grams, and most, if not all, of this should be monosaturated or polyunsaturated fat. You can achieve this by eating more vegetables, fruits and cereal grains, egg whites, complex carbohydrates, such as grains and legumes and nonfat products. Fortunately, over the last few years, nonfat food substitutes have become more readily available in supermarkets. You can even buy nonfat desserts and cheeses! In his recommended diet, Ornish eliminates caffeine and other stimulants as well as fish and fish oils. However, some dietitians believe that fish contain a fatty acid (omega-3) that may actually lower low-density lipoproteins (LDL, the "bad" kind).

To help you develop new eating habits and food tastes, develop new ways of cooking. Substitute lemon juice or a good brand of balsamic vinegar for the oils used in salad dressing. Sauté your vegetables in water, wine, or vegetable broth rather than oil. In recipes calling for cream, substitute nonfat milk or milk powder. Instead of eating ice cream, develop a taste for pure fruit sorbets. In *Dr. Dean Ornish's Program for Reversing Heart Disease*, there are many tasty recipes, and with a little imagination you might dream up many creative ways to eat really tasty nonfat foods.

Invitations to parties or dinners sometimes expose you to foods higher in fat and calories than you might like. One way to deal with such situations is to have a nonfat snack before you leave your home. Don't go famished; that way you can control what you eat or decide to pass up.

When you eat out, obtaining heart-healthy food can be a challenge, but is not impossible. Try enlisting the help of the person who serves you, and be gently insistent on obtaining what you need and want. Remember, restaurateurs depend on your patronage, waiters and waitresses on your largesse; they usually want to please and serve you. If you must eat protein, at least choose the foods with the lowest levels of saturated fat, such as fish or chicken, broiled or grilled rather than fried or sautéed; vegetables steamed or microwaved and served without butter or margarine; salads dressed with lemon or balsamic vinegar; potatoes served without butter or sour cream; coffee or tea served with skim or nonfat milk (I sometimes carry a small flask of skim milk with me when I eat out); fresh fruit or sorbet for dessert. Don't be fooled by those little hearts next to certain items on the menu. Even when the menu tells you that the item is prepared following American Heart Association (AHA) guidelines, remember that such guidelines are for the general public, not persons who already have evidence of atherosclerosis. AHA still believes that the total fat intake should be about 30 percent of one's diet. Many cardiologists are now saying that that figure is much too high and would recommend that it be cut down closer to 10 percent, even for the general public. One problem with maintaining a healthy diet is that there is too much public emphasis on calories and watching your weight—and too little on food designed to keep your coronary arteries (or the substitutes you obtained in bypass surgery) open rather than clogged. Society is supportive if you want to look good on the outside, but little support is given if you want your coronary arteries to stay healthy. It is absolutely essential that the bypass graduate take charge of and responsibility for what goes into his or her body. This isn't always easy, but with a positive attitude, healthy eating becomes a natural routine and part of a healthy lifestyle.

REHABILITATION AND EXERCISE

An essential aspect of maintaining your cardiac health is regular exercise. Exercise is both good for your heart and helps you control your weight. It also contributes to lowering your blood cholesterol levels. Ask your doctor about such programs and the kinds of exercises you should do.

Many medical centers where bypass surgery is performed also offer cardiac rehabilitation programs for persons who have had heart attacks and/or angioplasty and bypass operations. These programs are usually conducted by specially trained nurses, physical therapists, and other health personnel and include exercise programs as well as educational activities designed to inform the participant about the maintenance of his or her cardiac health. The bypass graduate, in particular, has an opportunity to meet others who have gone through similar experiences and who may be dealing with parallel problems of health maintenance. The social interactions that gradually develop among the program leaders and participants can play a major role in fostering healing and health.

Phase I of rehabilitation (rehab for short) for the person who has had bypass surgery generally begins while the patient is still in the hospital and consists of stretching and breathing exercises as well as brief walking exercises. Phase II is offered to bypass graduates after they have been discharged from the hospital.

The initial involvement with Phase II of a rehab program will probably require that you retake a stress treadmill test about six weeks after the surgery. The treadmill test may be conducted at the same site where, perhaps only a few weeks earlier, you first received your diagnosis of CAD. It should be expected that your associations with that site may not be positive and that you may have considerable anxiety about what the test will show. If the surgery was successful, however, your heart has been revascularized, and passing the treadmill test will probably be a breeze. Consider it a rite of passage to health.

A Phase II program generally involves supervised exercises, including a warm-up period of stretching and walking, aerobics designed to increase your heart rate to a target zone that has been previously determined on the basis of your treadmill results. Following the aerobic exercises, there is a cool-down period in which your heart rate and blood pressure return to baseline levels. Your heart rate is generally monitored closely in this phase of rehab.

In Phase III, if you continue with the rehab program, you do your own monitoring of your pulse rate and you have a wider variety of exercises to choose from. If you leave the rehab program, you need to choose whether or not to continue to exercise. If you want to maintain your cardiac health, there is only one choice to make: to continue in some regular exercise program. If you hate to exercise, join an exercise group. With social support, exercise becomes easier. Remember, physical exercise is one of the major keys to the maintenance of the gains bypass surgery provides.

Exercise also has a positive psychological impact. A heart attack, the diagnosis of CAD, and bypass surgery all tend to erode a person's confidence in his or her own body. One of the psychological purposes of exercise is to help restore that confidence or to build it if it wasn't there before. Exercise accomplishes this because one can see and experience the increasing effects of one's efforts over time.

Confidence in one's body also comes about from gaining greater understanding of how it functions, what it needs, how it communicates those needs, and how one's mind and body work together. Many persons, particularly after emergency bypass surgery, are motivated to read about how the body works, and to attend lectures dealing with various health problems such as how to eat right and how to reduce stress. These are positive attempts at mastering the bypass experience.

MANAGING STRESS

Most physicians advise patients who have had a heart attack or bypass surgery to reduce the stresses in their lives. Learning to relax, dealing with problems calmly, avoiding situations and persons that upset you, setting priorities, and so on are all good counsel. However, you cannot always avoid stressful situations since life is all too full of such circumstances. How you dealt with stresses in the past may need to be reexamined and changed so that your approach to such situations becomes more effective. There are multiple ways to deal with unavoidable stress, and some have already been described in Chapter 3. Such mind-body techniques as Progressive Relaxation, meditation, visualization, and so on are frequently taught in stress management programs to help you cope with stress more effectively. All of these techniques work because it is impossible to be tense and relaxed simultaneously. Your body will almost inevitably respond to mental images of mortal danger differently from a peaceful image of a lake ringed by trees and mountains. Responding to an image of danger, your endocrine system may begin to mobilize for fight-or-flight reactions, which will increase your heart rate, and your muscles will also tense as you ready yourself for action. The mental image of the peaceful scene, on the other hand, will promote an overall relaxation of your body.

In the book *Dr. Dean Ornish's Program for Reversing Heart Disease,* an entire chapter is devoted to various stress management techniques, many of which are illustrated and easy to follow. I strongly recommend any combination of these techniques to bypass graduates to manage the stresses in their lives. As with exercise, daily practice of stress-reducing procedures generally brings the greatest benefit.

DEALING WITH ANGER AND HOSTILITY

In research on the relationship between stress and heart disease, feelings of anger and hostility have emerged as factors believed to promote CAD. In effecting lifestyle changes after bypass surgery, the management of these feelings should receive special priority.

Recent data suggest that unexpressed anger may be even more harmful to your health than cigarette smoking, obesity, and a high-fat diet. Several long-term studies show that persons who scored high on hostility scales on personality tests at age twenty-five had a five times greater risk of being dead by age fifty than persons who scored low on such scales. It has been shown that women who at age eighteen answered test questions in a way that suggested they would suppress their anger were three times more likely to die within the next two decades than women who did not harbor such feelings. Longitudinal research has also shown that in contrast to persons who scored low on hostility scales, high scorers tended to have higher levels of low-density lipoproteins (the so-called bad form of cholesterol) and low levels of high-density lipoproteins (the good form of cholesterol).

The ancient Greeks understood the connection between anger and heart disease. The words *anger* and *angina* share a common root, *anchone* (a constriction or squeezing), and are associated with such words as *anguish* and *angst*. When the anger we feel comes from a sense of having been injured or mistreated, we frequently feel a desire to fight back or to harm the person we feel has injured us. For many individuals, these feelings and their accompanying vengeful thoughts are not permitted to enter consciousness. They are repressed, pushed into the unconscious recesses of our minds, often coming out in physical and physiological reactions, usually below our level of awareness. Presumably, this is one of the ways anger and hostility promote the chain of events leading to the buildup of plaque in our coronary arteries.

It should be reiterated that anger in itself may not be particularly harmful to one's self and to one's health. It may be the *quality* of the anger that distinguishes what may or may not be involved in promoting CAD. When anger has a bitter, unremitting, chronically festering quality to it and/or is rarely if ever appropriately externalized, it probably promotes the endocrine and other physiological events that lead to atherosclerosis.

Here are some pointers for dealing with anger. *First, when you are angry, acknowledge that you're angry.* This is not to say that you should punch out that scoundrel who backed into your brand-new car. It does mean that, in the privacy of your own space, you should acknowledge to yourself that you are infuriated and feel like doing something drastic to get even. Such private feelings and thoughts do no harm to anyone. Remember, thinking about how angry you are and acting it out are very, very different behaviors. The first step in dealing with angry feelings is to label them for what they are.

Second, when you find yourself behaving in a way that agitates you and starts to raise your blood pressure, stop and ask why you are reacting that way. You may find that you have a good answer to that question. For example, you may be late for an important meeting and that's why you are furious at the slowpoke in the car in front of you. If you do not have a good answer to the question or cannot come up with one, stop doing whatever you are doing to work yourself up and slow down your actions and your breathing. Tell yourself that you do not have to continue what you are doing. It's no good for you. It's no good for your health. Talk to yourself and calm yourself down and thus take conscious charge of your behavior.

Third, ask yourself what is making you so angry. At whom are you angry? Anger that is focused is easier to deal with than anger that is general and unfocused. Narrowing down the target of your anger generally makes it easier to think about what you might do to either express or control your feelings.

Fourth, assess how angry you are. Anger comes in many shapes and forms along a spectrum of annoyance, irritation, indignation, wrath, ire, rage, fury. Identify how angry you are. If necessary, use a ten-point scale and tell yourself you are such and such a number. Ask yourself whether the degree of your reaction is appropriate to the situation. Generally, it is stronger than it needs to be. Try to change your feelings to lower that number even just one point.

Fifth, decide in your mind what you want to do with your anger. Sometimes all you want is for someone to listen to your feelings. Talk about these feelings to someone you know will understand. You might want to take some appropriate action so that your anger is used in some constructive way. Writing a letter of protest, telling the person who is the cause of your anger how you feel and why you feel that way, and other such actions help to convert emotions into appropriate behavior and are effective ways of dealing with feelings that tend to occupy your thoughts and "eat away" at you.

Sixth, if talking things out and other appropriate responses fail to diminish your feelings of anger, seek professional help from someone with experience in this area.

THE LONG-TERM IMPACT OF BYPASS SURGERY

As recovery proceeds, you will no longer feel like a patient; you will feel more and more normal. Keep in mind, though, that in the eyes and minds of others, you may now be viewed as fragile. You might hear this in the subtle inflection of a friend's voice as she inquires how you are doing and how you are feeling. It reflects her caring as well as her concern about you. On the other hand, some "patients" report that they feel upset or insulted that others see them as being frail when they themselves feel more vital and vigorous than they have felt in years. You will need to maintain enormous patience in such situations.

Your self-image may also undergo alteration, even though you may feel stronger and more capable of physical exertion than you did before the surgery. You may begin to image yourself internally as being brittle or especially vulnerable insofar as your health is concerned. If others seem to "see" you as frail or changed, you may begin to think that perhaps there is some truth in their perceptions. Such thoughts may interact with your own tendency to interpret small, subtle internal and external states as being more important than they really are.

If you have lived your life based on the beliefs that you are immortal and invulnerable to the aging process, there's nothing like bypass surgery to give you a sense of reality. Undoubtedly, for some this is an intense narcissistic injury; that is, discovering that you are only human may be experienced as a slap in the face, an insult. This realization may lead to a number of psychological problems, not the least of which may be depression. Fortunately, most of us do not base our lives on such unrealistic underpinnings, and thus we have greater resilience to cope with the life challenges of the postoperative period.

Returning to work and other accustomed activities after bypass surgery is often welcomed as a sign of increasing normality. But the entire experience often makes bypass graduates aware that their interests, energy, and perseverance may not be what they once were.

Changes in your interests and in the direction of your work are not unusual after bypass surgery. For some, travel and other pleasurable activities may gain priority over work-related ones. Many bypass graduates cut back on work-related efforts, take retirement, and reduce other responsibilities for the sake of a more easygoing life. When these changes are made consciously and are experienced as a matter of choice, they are generally handled effectively over time. If, on the other hand, you feel such changes have been "forced" upon you, as for example, in the case of a client whose spouse was so traumatized by his bypass surgery that she insisted he retire and stay at home, adverse psychological consequences may follow.

When Things Don't Go Right

Not all bypass surgeries have a positive outcome. Undoubtedly, death or a debilitating stroke during or immediately following the procedure is the worst-case scenario. For the survivors, the emptiness of the loss of the person is experienced in full force. On average, for all patients undergoing bypass surgery the overall mortality rate is about 2 percent; patients who have the procedure on an elective basis tend to have a risk of about 1 percent.

Some 5 to 10 percent of patients experience postoperative complications. These range from the serious (for example, a heart attack or stroke) to the annoying (infections). In general, the person's preoperative health and life habits appear to be a major contributor to complications following bypass surgery. Smokers, for example, have a higher risk for lung complications after such surgery since their lungs are already damaged by smoking. Also, obese individuals have a tendency to develop circulatory complications such as leg clots, since their circulatory systems may already be compromised by their excess weight. Sometimes an artery that feeds the brain becomes blocked, perhaps by a small blood clot released in the course of the surgery, leading to a transient ischemial accident (TIA), a temporary condition, or to a permanent stroke. Also, because the heart is manipulated during the surgery, portions of the heart may become irritated, which may lead to problems in pumping the blood and/or maintaining a steady heart rate after the surgery. These problems are generally treated with drugs. Infections of the wound in the sternum or the leg may sometimes lead to fevers and are often treated with antibiotics.

When problems do occur during or after surgery, they often slow down or retard the process of recuperation. This, in turn, may have negative psychological consequences. If the patient has felt that he or she is recovering rapidly from the surgery and a setback occurs, it may promote a sense of discouragement. Medical personnel and significant others need to remain sensitive to the patient's needs during these periods, accentuating the positive and giving lots of encouragement, rewarding each small recuperative step, and providing perspective. Remind the patient that recuperation isn't always a linear upward process. Like the tide, it tends to have an ebb and flow, a back and forth. But no matter what the rate of recovery is, over time the patient will probably find that he or she has increasing capacities and tends to feel better. Also, localize the impact of setbacks. If the leg wound is not healing properly, remind the patient that it's only the leg that needs a little more time to heal, whereas the *person* is getting better and better each day.

The significant other of the patient has enormous psychological tasks to accomplish in the immediate postsurgical period, but this is another chapter.

SUGGESTED READING

Angier, N. 1990. Anger can ruin more than your day. *The New York Times,* Dec. 13, p. B1–B7.

Anon. 1988. *After Your Heart Attack*. Daly City, CA: Krames Publ.

Cohn, K., D. Duke, and J. A. Madrid. 1979. *Coming Back*. Reading, Mass.: Addison-Wesley Publ. Co.

Horovitz, E. 1988. *Heart Beat*. Los Angeles: Health Trend Publ.

Ornish, D. 1990. *Dr. Dean Ornish's Program for Reversing Heart Disease*. New York: Random House.

Ornish, D. 1993. *Eat More, Weigh Less*. New York: HarperCollins. (For the experienced cook; great recipes.)

Schlesinger, S. 1994. *500 Fat-Free Recipes*. New York: Villard Books. (Less interesting recipes, but much easier to make.)

Superko, H. R., and R. M. Krauss. 1994. Coronary artery regression. Convincing evidence for the benefit of aggressive lipoprotein management. *Circulation* 90: 1056–1069.

S I X

. . . .

A SPOUSE'S PERSPECTIVE

W hen your husband, wife, or significant other is required to undergo bypass surgery—any major surgery for that matter—you know that you will have to face many challenges. You will also feel anxious, perhaps frightened. You may have to face the possibility of having him or her die or left an invalid as a result of the operation. You probably understand that he or she may require considerable caretaking and that your "normal" life may be completely disrupted. Also, you probably know how he or she handles anxiety under stress, and that may not be something you look forward to.

Your life, like your partner's, will be changed, perhaps in many unanticipated ways. You may feel afraid and unable to share your feelings with your partner because he or she has enough to deal with already and you do not wish to burden him or her further. You may have to make decisions for which you may not be prepared, requiring you to gather facts, information, and advice, both independently and together with your partner. You too have a lot to deal with, and you may have few ears into which to pour your complaints, confusions, and consternations. Perhaps this chapter will help.

Since, at the present time, men have bypass surgery more

frequently than women, in a ratio of three to one, the average spouse or significant other is most likely to be a woman. As greater attention is paid to the incidence of heart disease among women (as with men, heart disease is the number one cause of death among women) the situation in the future may change. However, the discussion in this chapter will focus on the female partner as the spouse and her male mate as the patient.

FEARS

Underlying much of the spouse's anxiety is the threat that her mate might die during or as a result of the surgery. No one I know, even persons who hate their mates, wants to experience this loss and be left bereaved. Every spouse I ever talked to professionally, excepting those who were incredible deniers, had had thoughts about their mate's death, considered its possibility, and to greater or lesser extent dealt with the anxieties it raised, generally by preparing themselves for that possibility.

The average mortality rate as the result of bypass surgery appears to be between 1 and 2 percent; relatively low. But, if it's your mate, that figure can seem unacceptably large, and understandably so.

Statisticians generally deal with groups rather than with specific individuals. The rest of humanity deals with statistics in a more normal, personal way—that is, our primary focus is on ourselves and the people we feel close to. Thus, from our perspective, one to two deaths per hundred doesn't seem so small and is almost invariably frightening to contemplate. Your mate might be that one. This difference in perspective is a reality that comes up over and over again between physicians and patients.

The solace we try to give ourselves is twofold. We try to focus on the fact that 98 to 99 persons out of 100 *do* make it through the surgery. There is comfort in that. Our mate has a strong chance of making it. Also, we recognize that we need faith—faith in God, faith in our surgeons, faith in our ourselves, and faith that the outcome will be successful. We do this to control our fears and to keep our anxieties from overwhelming us, and this is our major task at this moment. Most spouses exert this control successfully.

TASKS AND EMOTIONAL DEMANDS

The spouse is likely to be under considerable stress in the periods before, during, and immediately after surgery, and this stress may affect her own physical and psychological health. It is imperative that the spouse maintain her own health during this period if she wants to be a helpmate to the patient. This may mean finding ways to defuse the anxieties and fears that may arise by personal management (e.g., meditation), talking it out with friends and/or professionals, etc. Sometimes having a realistic sense of what is happening and what to expect in the days and weeks ahead helps the spouse manage her feelings.

Generally, in the initial stages of the bypass process, the spouse tends to be very supportive of the patient and attentive to the latter's needs. However, when it becomes clear that the patient is "out of the woods," the spouse often allows the feelings that may have been suppressed during the period of crisis to emerge in force. Intense feelings of anger toward the patient for how he has been living his life—his diet, lack of exercise, etc.—and for putting her through such frightening, anxiety-provoking times often are expressed. Also, as the patient returns to full functioning, the spouse may allow her feelings of fatigue and depletion to surface. This may be expressed her becoming depressed and sending out messages that "Now it's my turn to get some caretaking."

The spouse may need to make enormous life changes as a result of her mate's surgery. These changes might include taking on new and unaccustomed roles and responsibilities in the home and workplace. Many wives of individuals who have had bypass surgery attempt to learn new ways of cooking so as to provide low-cholesterol, low-fat meals for their husbands. Few husbands appreciate the amount of time, energy, planning, and emotional investment their wives make in this regard.

The emotional demands bypass surgery places on spouses in many ways are greater than those on patients. Frequently, their emotional needs become subordinated to those of the patient, especially just prior to and after surgery. They often need to defer the expression of their feelings for long periods of time in the service of appearing optimistic, happy, and satisfied for the sake of their children and/or mate while inwardly they may feel very alone, despairing, and deeply unhappy. They may also "go along" with decisions and plans that they know are either not sensible or would only add further emotional burdens on them, all for the sake of others.

COPING WITH THE DIAGNOSIS OF CAD

When the diagnosis of CAD is first made, the spouse as well as the patient generally becomes upset. However, the latter often has some task or tasks to accomplish—for example, taking medications, arranging for further tests, doctor's appointments, and the like. The spouse, on the other hand, because her role is less

clear than the patient's, under these circumstances may feel helpless and such feelings may in turn promote catastrophic thinking.
Thoughts of loss or the possibility of loss may surface and may
generate considerable anxiety and fear.

Not only must the spouse manage her own emotions, but also
she almost invariably needs to monitor her mate's emotional
state and modify her own reactions accordingly. If the patient is
anxious or "falling apart," the spouse feels compelled to remain
cool and calm. Someone has to hold it together.

Some patients withdraw into themselves, leaving others
around them wondering what they're feeling and thinking. In
the absence of verbal feedback, the spouse is liable to slip into
morbid fantasizing, catastrophic thinking, and the like. If, on the
other hand, the patient is calm and seemingly unconcerned,
going about his activities as if nothing unusual is going on, this
too might raise the spouse's levels of anxiety. Sometimes the
spouse may just find it easier to join the patient in denying the
magnitude of the problem to keep her own anxiety under control. If such denial leads to procrastination about necessary medical decisions, such as, for example, further tests or surgery, the
couple is playing cardiac "Russian roulette," hardly a situation
that will ultimately reduce their levels of stress.

The fact that men and women often react differently to stress,
utilizing differing defenses and styles of coping, often translates
into women's carrying a disproportionate share of the emotional
burden in a family. For example, when it becomes apparent that
bypass surgery is necessary, the children and friends may need to
be notified and such tasks often fall to women in the family.
When friends and relatives are notified about the surgery, they
tend to react strongly to such news and project their own anxieties and fears about the patient; the spouse may be required to
protect the patient from such reactions.

The desire to protect a spouse is a common reaction. However, there are limits as to how much protection one can provide, and this needs to be recognized and acknowledged. One's partner is not a child and should be able, even under stress, to take self-protective actions. The spouse needs to tread a fine line, on one hand of not infantilizing the patient but, on the other, not exposing him to the fears, negative thoughts, and sometimes thoughtless comments of others.

In addition, the spouse has to deal with the ongoing ups and downs of the patient. In the period between the diagnosis of CAD and the surgery, the patient may undergo a subtle transformation, not always positive. For example, one spouse described her husband as follows:

> B. was already acquiring his father's gait. Whereas in the past his pace would have been brisk and lively, now it was measured and careful. His whole being seemed consumed with fear. I felt it in his touch, heard it in his voice, and saw it in his eyes. He talked about the impact the doctor's instructions had on him following the treadmill test. He was terrified when told that he could no longer pick up a heavy object, walk up steep hills, travel in a carefree style, or exert himself in any fashion.

Experiencing these changes in the self-perception of the patient perforce affects the spouse's perceptions as well, and reinforces the sense that loss may be just around the corner.

Under stress and in the face of crisis, couples tend to either pull together to cooperate and work as a team or fall upon one another with accusations, antagonisms, blaming, arguments, and the like, externalizing their inner anxieties. For troubled couples, the presurgical period may be one of hell and may require the intervention of an outside professional. Fortunately, most couples have the capacity to control their anxieties and to greater or lesser degree work together to prepare for the surgery. The need to do so is enormous. For example, much information may need to be obtained and digested in preparation for the surgery and there are multiple decisions to be made. By acting as a team, couples can get through this preparatory work and focus on the true goal of surgery, which is to help the patient rebuild his or her health.

COPING WITH THE PRESURGICAL PERIOD

One of the central issues some couples need to face in the pre-surgical period is who will make the decision about having the surgery. Is it only up to the patient or does the spouse have a say also? And if the spouse has some input, how much and when? An important role the spouse might play in the presurgical period is that of an advocate to assist the patient in thinking through his or her options. By acting as a sounding board for the patient's thoughts, a spouse can point out options he might have missed.

One couple I spoke to described their situation as follows:

> D. and I agreed at the onset that this was to be his decision. He had to make a choice about his life, and that decision had to be made freely and intelligently. When he became depressed or defeated after a medical interview, it was my role to remind him of all the counterarguments, to argue the opposing side, so that

he would have to become engaged again in the debate.
It wasn't difficult for me to take the opposing position,
for it closely represented my true opinion at that time.
I did not favor his having the surgery. On the other
hand, I had to respect that this was his life and his decision.

Some patients like to go it alone. From his perspective this
may help him to contain his anxiety. But, this may leave the
spouse and others cut out from the process of thinking and decision-making, which in turn may raise the spouse's own anxieties
and fears. This fact should be pointed out to the patient and ways
to open up the solo thinking process should be explored. One
way the spouse might accomplish this is to stay as informed as
possible about the available procedures and options. If you want
your opinion to be heard, you need to stay abreast of and possibly ahead on the issues with which your partner is dealing. To
maintain credibility, the spouse needs to take a parallel journey
to that of her mate.

One woman put it this way:

> I couldn't assist S. on his journey [preparing for the
> surgery] without taking a similar journey with him in
> my own way. Each day I meditated on his imminent
> voyage, accepting its reality and sensing what he was
> about to experience. That helped me to better under-
> stand and appreciate his thoughts and feelings. It gave
> me insight into what he would need in order to sup-
> port and enhance his experience.

Many spouses accompanied their mates when they went for
appointments with surgeons and actively stayed on top of the

information they were gathering as a couple. This cooperation gives the couple the sense that they are operating as a team, thus reducing the feeling of helplessness many tend to feel in this presurgical period.

Although the ultimate decision about the surgery is generally the patient's, the spouse may have her own opinions and thoughts. Some wives prefer that their husbands not have the surgery, hoping that their mate will choose a less drastic way of treating his condition. Some are wary about sharing their thoughts with their mates, others are suspicious about their own motivations and are aware that sometimes their own fears of surgery and other factors are operating. Almost every spouse I have spoken with had to take cues from her mate. For example, one woman said:

> I had to take my cues from Jack. This was his illness, his life, his decision, not mine. And his decision would be based on his understanding of the risks he was willing to take.

Another woman, when asked how she felt about her husband's decision to have bypass surgery, responded:

> I knew that he was doing what was right for him. Nonetheless, I felt a twinge of disappointment. All along I wished that he would be willing to try to reverse the coronary artery occlusions without surgery. That would be my choice. But it wasn't for him and I couldn't impose what was right for me on him. I had to force myself to comprehend the choice from his perspective, taking into consideration the type of person he is, the way he thinks, his motivations, and so

on. It took me about a day to work it out in my mind and to appreciate the world from his perspective. I knew I had to accept his decision.

H E L P I N G   Y O U R   M A T E   P R E P A R E   F O R   S U R G E R Y

Spouses can also play an active role in helping the patient prepare psychologically for the days ahead. Suggest that you and he set time aside each day before the surgery just to talk. Disconnect the phone and ignore the doorbell for thirty minutes or so and simply talk and listen to one another. Perhaps meditate together and share the thoughts and feelings that arise in such meditations. Give your mate a massage, help him relax, say soothing things, allow yourselves to feel close to one another and to others who are close to you.

Do not assume that your spouse will react in his usual way. Remember that he is probably under stress and is feeling vulnerable. Thus, do not be surprised if old defensive, guarded stances dissolve almost overnight and that he becomes more emotionally available during this period. When your mate is relaxed, help him put words to his fears and anxieties. Listen. Do not give him false reassurances. Just listen and understand. He may need to make peace with you and others about long-standing conflicts and may require your support during this time to do so.

Help him image the trip to the hospital, the admission, the first day, the surgery itself, the immediate postsurgical period. Help him image his life afterward, the changes in his life with you that you may both dream about. Set time aside each day, even several times a day if possible, to meditate and to visualize the surgery and the postsurgical period.

One of the essential pieces of advice I would give to spouses is to be scrupulous about caring for their own health. When the patient sees that his mate is taking care of herself, it gives him the feeling that there is someone out there on whom he can depend and rely. Conversely, if the spouse is careless or negligent about, or inattentive to, her person or her health, the patient generally has little or no confidence that the spouse will be supportive as a helpmate. Almost invariably this feeling will create anxiety for the patient, and make it difficult for him to prepare adequately for the surgery.

The fact that the spouse is also under considerable stress may compromise her immune system and increase her vulnerability to infections and the like. Thus, the spouse needs to make extraordinary efforts to stay healthy. In this regard, procedures such as meditation to reduce tension and stress may be invaluable.

For some insights into the spouse's role during the hospital period, you could refer to my wife's diary in Chapter 4.

COPING IN THE POSTSURGICAL PERIOD

Once the patient comes home after surgery, new challenges arise. One of the initial tasks the spouse faces is setting up the home so that her mate can be cared for during the first weeks after surgery. If there are many steps to climb in your home, it might be easier to set up a bed on the first floor. Also, your mate will probably require your assistance to get out of bed. Thus you'll need to set up a way for him to communicate with you when he needs help.

The second challenge is learning when and how to help the patient. During the first week or so back home, the patient's needs will change from day to day, depending on his energy that day and other factors. His capacity one day may not be there the day after. On one hand, you do not want to underestimate his ability and thus possibly compromise his self-esteem. On the other hand, you do not want to overestimate his ability, thereby leading to experiences of defeat, which in turn might lead to depression. Your role in this period requires a balancing act (again!) based on the feedback you receive from your mate about his perception of his own energy and the degree to which he is willing and able to push himself. How should you treat him, as a sick person or as a healthy man who, at this point, needs special attention? It doesn't pay to make decisions for him about these matters since only he knows the answer to that question.

Keep in mind that although your mate's physical condition may compromise his self-sufficiency, thus making him dependent on you, it does not compromise his self-awareness and his need for psychological independence. The latter requires your respect, support, and understanding. How you manage this issue independent of all other factors may determine how quickly your mate recuperates and becomes normally functional.

Perhaps a useful model to keep in mind is the following. The surgery requires the patient to regress psychologically—that is, to function in a way more appropriate to an earlier stage of maturation. During the surgery he is totally regressed, almost like a fetus whose survival depends wholly on an external source of nourishment. Immediately after the surgery he is, developmentally speaking, at about the level of an infant. Almost every need—nutrition, hygiene, etc.—has to be taken care of by the adults around him. When he emerges from the anesthesia, he is similar psychologically to a young child (see Chapter 4). By the time he comes home from the hospital, he probably has the ability to walk and communicate, but many aspects of his functioning are not at a mature adult level. He still requires adult supervision and caretaking. His moods may be determined by his energy, and when that wanes he may become irritable and cranky. His appetite may also regress to a childlike level. He, like a young child, may be interested in eating only simple foods, unspiced, such as pasta or potatoes, rather than poultry or fish and his usual exotic fare. Approach it as if you are feeding and dealing with a five- or six-year-old child.

Like all children, he has a need for autonomy and self-sufficiency. If he does not have opportunities to learn that he can do things for himself, his developmental progress will be impeded. Thus, like a good parent, you need to balance your need to have him dependent on your ministrations (because you may derive pleasure and satisfaction from such activities, or because it is quicker and easier for you to do it yourself) and his need for independence.

Just as we all have needs for autonomy, we also have conscious and unconscious needs to be dependent. We often enjoy it when others take care of us. Thus, for some patients the sick role may be difficult to relinquish. Similarly, some spouses have difficulty letting go of their caretaking role and as a consequence give their mates the message that they are far sicker and less capable than they actually are. Both situations can lead to invalidism of the patient and the development of a dysfunctional relationship between the spouse and mate that may become a prescription for depression in one or both of them.

By the second day home, it is advisable to establish a daily rhythm. This gives your mate a sense of control over his activities and a growing feeling that he is getting back in charge of his life. A sense of rhythm is also useful for the spouse, since it allows her to know when she can take time out for her own personal activities. Encourage your mate to wake early, get out of bed, shave, shower, and dress. Perhaps after breakfast and a short rest, go out for a walk with him. Encourage him to read even if his attention span (like that of a child) is short. Limit his television watching just as you would a child's. One alternative to reading and television is listening to books on audiotape. This too ought to be limited, since wearing headphones promotes a sense of social isolation and withdrawal and this could induce a depressive mood.

Encourage your mate to continue meditating and, if possible, help him to do so. The focus at this point is on healing and visualizing a healthy future life.

Meditate yourself. Visualize what your life will be like in the weeks, months, and years ahead. Visualize how you will obtain what you need for yourself and how you will find joy and satisfaction with (or without) your mate.

Encourage friends to visit and/or to take your mate out for walks. Social interactions are a preventive for depression—it's just good medicine. The need to feel that others care is important for both you and your mate. On the other hand, be aware of the fact that not all your friends or relatives are able to deal well with illness or with a recuperating patient and that the latter will probably be drained by a visit from such persons. A timely intervention on your part in these situations would be appreciated all around.

DEALING WITH YOUR MATE AFTER SURGERY

As the patient recovers, he will probably have to face the fact that his body is scarred and that his sense of bodily integrity and wholeness has been undermined. The surgery changes one's body image. In particular, the perceived sense of personal power associated with one's chest region often tends to be compromised, creating a sense of helplessness in that body area. Such feelings are further exacerbated by the patient's inability to move from the lying to the sitting or standing position without assistance. Also, the patient may feel repulsed by what he sees in the mirror and might expect that his spouse will have similar feelings. This may lead to difficulties in achieving intimacy in the relationship with the spouse.

The spouse should be aware that the patient may be extremely sensitive about being touched in the chest region. Many patients tend to turn away or recoil from the touch of their spouses and some raise their arms to "protect" themselves when approached, as if they were being assaulted. These are attempts to avert further injury and pain.

Since a negative body image may lower your mate's self-esteem, which, in turn, might promote or exacerbate depressive feelings, it might be prudent for the spouse to intervene as soon as possible to reassure him that he is not ugly or repulsive. Perhaps one of the most effective ways of dealing with this situation, for both of you, is to use desensitization measures by means of gentle massage. In this process you would, over time, repeatedly touch your mate's chest, thus desensitizing its appearance for you and simultaneously conveying to your mate that he and his chest are not ugly or repulsive. The massages would also help him learn that he can allow his chest to be touched without fear that it will lead to injury or pain. In short, it helps your mate unlearn behavior associated with the trauma of the surgery and relearn more adaptive responses associated with tenderness and safety.

The Massage Is the Message

Start out by gently applying a rich solution of body lotion, first to your mate's back, a less sensitive area than the chest. Only at a pace acceptable to him the lotion is then gently applied to the chest, moving from the intact areas slowly toward the scarred area with very gentle massage movements. The legs should also be massaged, first the "good" leg and then, using an upward stroke (toward the heart), the "bad" leg. Massaging the leg from which the vein has been removed probably helps to reduce the edema and promotes an improved circulation.

Whatever the possible medical effects, massage simply feels good. Moreover, it tells your mate that you are not afraid to touch him and that you still find him lovable and desirable. Remember to remind both your mate and yourself that although the scar is now a part of him, it is only a part, not the whole of him.

The massages may also have the effect of bringing the two of you closer together in a more intimate way and allowing you to experience the pleasure of being a wife and companion again.

PICKING UP THE PIECES OF YOUR OWN LIFE

As it becomes clear that your mate is on his way to recovery, it becomes extremely important for you to resume your normal activities as soon as feasible. The patient may begin to feel guilty or like a burden if he sees you "sacrificing" your life for him, especially when he knows that he can largely take care of himself.

Re-entering your normal activities may prove to be another

challenge. Up to this point a great deal of your time and energy may have been centered on your mate and on the surgery. You may have become deeply involved with the situation, but now it may be time to begin to let go and move on. However, you may be wiped out by the emotionality of the past several days or weeks and the necessity of having to face yet another personal challenge may not exactly be welcome. The best advice is to go slowly, allowing time for the transition and not expecting miracles from yourself. The transitions involved in returning to work or other usual activities following a period of personal tumult almost invariably turn out to be far more demanding than most people realize.

Most spouses of bypass patients experience some form of post-surgical fatigue or letdown when their mates show signs of normality and recovery. They are exhausted and many try to hide that fact from their mate and others. But the fact is that although the surgeon has not operated on them, they often feel traumatized because they have had to "put out" a great deal of emotional energy, if for no other reason than to appear calm and collected for the sake of the patient and others. It takes a lot of energy to maintain a camouflage act.

Compared to the intensity and, perhaps, excitement of the period just before and after the surgery, the recovery period for the spouse often may be staid, uneventful, and relatively low-keyed. Activities that were part of your routine as a couple before the surgery may be gradually reinstated and resumed. This is an opportunity to re-identify yourself within the context of the larger arena of family, friends, community, work, etc. In other words, with the whole panoply of your attachments and interests. Some couples take this period as an opportunity to take a vacation to some exotic or romantic locale as a means of restoring intimacy and redefining their relationship. It also provides the opportunity to reexperience one another as mates or partners rather than as nurse and patient.

The transition between the nurse and patient roles and new ones based on a foundation of health and full functioning requires the spouse to relinquish the degree of caregiving that has been established and to return to "normal" activities. The former patient, however, may have difficulty giving up the "sick" role and may interfere with the spouse's attempts to pick up the pieces of her life, consciously or otherwise continuing to place demands on her. It needs to be remembered she may feel exhausted and unable or unwilling to meet the former patient's demands. These feelings should be communicated to the mate as tactfully as possible and with words of encouragement, pointing out how much stronger or healthier he is, and that the time has come for him to reduce his demands.

One of the pitfalls in this postsurgical period is the wish on the part of both spouse and patient to obtain some reward or compensation for their efforts in the presurgical and surgical periods. This may be expressed in terms of further demands on the part of the patient, and possibly "Now it's my turn for nurturance and support" messages on the part of the spouse. Sometimes this latter message is conveyed in physical terms by the spouse's falling ill. In one case the wife of a man who had a heart attack and bypass surgery subsequently broke her leg. In another case the husband of a woman who just had bypass surgery had a heart attack soon after she came home from the hospital. Psychotherapists see similar situations so frequently it is difficult to believe they are all coincidental. If the feelings around these issues can be expressed verbally, it might help the couple to recognize and acknowledge their needs for attention and dependence without necessarily having to fulfill them on either side.

Many spouses have the satisfaction of knowing they have

played their part as a caregiver impeccably. But often they feel that the extent of their efforts has not been appreciated and the price they have paid physically and emotionally is unnoticed and unacknowledged. Mates need to be more attentive to their spouse's needs. Lacking that, spouses need to be more assertive in making their needs known. You have a right to have your needs met.

ASSESSING THE IMPACT OF THE SURGERY

Life sometimes changes dramatically for both patient and spouse after the dust settles. For one thing, the spouse may need to institute and maintain a new culinary low-fat and low- or no-cholesterol regimen. This may be very time-consuming, especially at the beginning when new cooking techniques, recipes, and menus need to be acquired. But on a deeper level, the spouse's life may feel fundamentally altered. She is now more conscious of the mate's mortality and the fragility of their life together. If the patient returns to old habits, such as smoking, consuming high-fat foods, and getting little or no exercise, the spouse may (inwardly or outwardly) become enraged because of her awareness that they may soon have to go through the trauma of heart attack and/or surgery again. And this time he may not make it through. Rather than investing their energies in trying to save their mates, some spouses turn toward their own latent strengths and to talents heretofore underutilized to find ways of assuring that their life will continue as comfortably as possible should their mate die. There is also the awareness that one cannot force one's mate to adopt life-affirming behavior; one can only control one's own actions.

Like the patient, the spouse may have to question the meaning and direction of her life after bypass surgery. Many have used this harrowing experience and its aftermath to effect major changes in their thinking and in their lives.

In my experience, the spouse of an individual who has undergone bypass surgery often has a very different perspective on the pre- and postsurgical events than the patient. In some ways it is more realistic and less defensive than that of the patient. For example, the postsurgical individual may not experience himself as being very different from the presurgical person. One man who had had a bypass two years earlier said in an upbeat way, "Yes, I'm still the same energetic man I was before." His wife, however, had a completely different viewpoint. She saw her husband as having far less energy and as tending to become depressed more easily and more frequently than he had before the surgery.

Before closing, it needs to be pointed out that bypass surgery also has an enormous impact on the patient's children. They too have had to face the fact that their parent(s) are not immortal and they may have had to take on unanticipated caregiving duties. Also, the children may have to deal with their own feelings of anger, disappointment, concern, and, last but not least, personal vulnerability that are aroused by the fact that their parent required bypass surgery.

It will take time to sort out and adjust to these new thoughts and roles. Patience, and taking time to communicate and listen, seem to be the key to getting through this often difficult transition.

SEVEN

· · · · · · · · · ·

MAKING SENSE OUT OF IT ALL

*Illness takes away parts of your life, but in doing so it gives
you the opportunity to choose the life you will lead, as opposed to living out the one you have simply accumulated over
the years.*

—ARTHUR W. FRANK

The heart has long been understood to function as something considerably more than a vascular pump. The language we
use often betrays understandings hidden from our conscious
awareness and exposes knowledge flowing from a source deep in
the recesses of the past that illuminates the meanings we give our
life experiences. Thus, the heart has come to be understood as
the center of understanding, emotion, and character in addition
to whatever physiological role it plays. In the Bible, God
punishes Pharaoh by closing or hardening his heart to reason,
compassion, and understanding. We speak of true emotion as
being *heartfelt*. A person who shows no feelings in circumstances
that commonly require emotional expression is called *heartless* or
cold-hearted. Loss is often experienced as *heartache*. Love is frequently depicted as a heart pierced by Cupid's arrow. The heart
is a metaphor for the human being and for the human condition.

In their book *Bypass: A Cardiologist Reveals What Every Patient
Needs to Know* (New York: Random House, 1985), Jonathan
Halperin and Richard Levine write:

Bypass surgery is a confrontation with one's mortality.
. . . Once someone has held your heart in his hand, its
beat will forever have new meaning. Anxiety, depression, fear, guilt, confusion, and lapses of memory—the
symptoms, some of which took root in the operating
room, comingle with each other and feed on life's ev-
eryday difficulties. Patients are robbed of their sense of
well-being or infused with self-doubt. Others cope
with the realization of having suddenly grown frail and
old. . . . Decades ago, before the era of open-heart
surgery, patients with diseased and malfunctioning
heart valves were consigned to live as invalids, and became known as cardiac cripples. Now it seems as
though bypass surgery, a cornerstone of medicine's
spectacular counterattack against coronary disease, is
creating a new generation of cripples.

I thought about this pessimistic assessment and my own experience as well as the experiences of clients and others I interviewed, and saw so little relevance of one to the other. Perhaps
Halperin and Levine are writing about individuals who have had
sudden heart attacks and nonelective bypass surgery, possibly
under nonoptimum conditions, and have emerged traumatized
by the entire set of experiences. But this is a limited perspective
at best.

Of course, one's heartbeat takes on new meaning. But does it
have to be one of inevitable loss, of being robbed of youth and
vitality, or of invalidism? Absolutely not.

One cannot always choose the challenges one will face during
one's lifetime. Some challenges are predictable, others not.
Some, such as career or parenthood, come as a result of choice.
Others, such as the death of a parent, are unwelcome but not

unexpected. Yet other challenges such as a heart attack and bypass surgery are often thrust upon us, also unwelcome and not of our choosing. But regardless of the turns our lives take, it is not the challenge that matters, but how we respond. A wise man once said, "We all fall on our faces. It's how we get up that makes all the difference."

No one would want to have bypass surgery if there were another way to treat their heart disease. But once this challenge is thrust upon you, a major choice arises: either to view it as a catastrophe or to view it as an unexpected opportunity for personal growth and enrichment.

Viewed as a catastrophe, heart bypass can lead to feelings of loss, of being robbed or cheated and humiliated. The "good life" has been taken away. The mental set established from this starting point is likely to lead to resistance toward and unpreparedness for the surgery. And what can you expect afterward? Growth from the experience? Lifestyle changes? Wisdom? Hardly. On the other hand, when viewed as an opportunity for growth, heart bypass opens many psychological doors.

There is a sense of joy and strength at having risen to a challenge and overcome an obstacle that comes with seeing bypass surgery as an opportunity for a recommitment to life and health. Rather than being left bereft and grieving for the past, you might emerge renewed and looking forward to an active, healthy future. Instead of self-doubt, you may have greater confidence arising from the fact that you have participated successfully in a heroic act of choice. Rather than emerging frail and senile, you may choose increased wisdom and a new, more realistic sense of self.

Possibly because it is an encounter with mortality, bypass surgery tends to make you more sensitive to and aware of your inner physical and psychological world. It opens you to inner dimensions that have been there all along but that you may not have been aware of or attuned to. Bypass graduates often find themselves evaluating and re-evaluating their lives, sorting through the inner attics and basements of memory and experience, rearranging, discarding, altering the careworn items, repairing the things that are frayed and tattered. Among the latter items are close relationships with friends and relatives that in the course of life become jaded, possibly taken for granted. After bypass surgery the quality of relationships with friends and relatives often undergoes a positive change—or so many alumni of this procedure report. Many of these changes occur because of the psychological impact on the patient and on others around him or her. Bypass surgery opens the heart to such change. It is no coincidence that bypass surgery is commonly called *open heart surgery*.

One of the most frequent comments you will hear from persons who have undergone bypass surgery is how often they remind themselves how precious life is. It is inevitable to think about this after major surgery. The surgery brings you face to face with mortality and the fact that life literally may hang by thin threads. As Saul Bellow wrote, "Death is the dark backing a mirror needs if we want to see anything"; the surgery gives you a glimpse of that end of life.

It is almost impossible not to reassess one's life following bypass surgery. What have you accomplished? To what do you want to devote the rest of your life? Most of us have postponed answering the tough questions about existence and our place in the scheme of the universe. After the surgery it isn't as easy to procrastinate because you are more aware of having brushed by the endpoint just a few weeks or months ago. For many there is much they still want to accomplish in their lives. But everything hinges on the maintenance of good health, which, in turn, requires a commitment to retain for as long as possible the gains of the surgery.

The surgery generally leaves you with a revascularized heart. In other words, the heart musculature, previously starved for nourishment and working inefficiently at best, now has a renewed source of oxygen-rich, nourishing blood. The heart is rejuvenated. For many, this opens the way to a more active, vital way of life. For all, it requires important choices.

LIFE CHOICES

As a bypass graduate, you have one of three choices. You can: (1) Attempt to put the experience as far behind you as possible and resume the life you led before the surgery; (2) Live as a cardiac cripple; or (3) Attempt to use the experience to create something new for yourself.

Returning to the Past

One obvious choice open to us following bypass surgery is to return to the life habits that brought us to the surgeon's door. This, largely, is a life based on denial.

There is a poster hanging near the treadmill apparatus at my rehab center showing a photograph of a man with a bloated beer belly hanging obscenely over his belt. The caption accompanying the photograph reads: "Millions of Americans are suffering from a major health problem—Denial." There is enormous truth to this. We live our lives with self-delusion regarding many of our life habits, particularly around the treatment of our bodies. It is as if we feel we can live unhealthily and abuse our bodies with impunity.

One of the tragedies of our culture is that there is relatively little support for health-promoting behaviors. It took many decades of research and advertising campaigns to draw sufficient public attention to the effects of cigarette smoking on the development of cardiovascular disease and lung cancer to allow the appearance of warning labels on tobacco products. It is also known that passive exposure to the cigarette smoke of others increases the risk for lung cancer. Yet, how many restaurants and other business establishments do you know that have adequately separate smoker and nonsmoker sections?

Similar observations can be made about the fat and cholesterol content of food. We live in a culture that relishes fat and cholesterol and consumes it in copious quantities. Some estimates suggest that nearly 40 to 50 percent of the average American caloric intake consists of fat. We are surrounded by it and encouraged against our better instincts to get that dessert on the special dessert menu to top off that already high-calorie, fat-rich meal.

It takes enormous self-control not to eat fat-rich foods. There are few social or societal controls supporting a resolve not to eat a fat-rich diet. Certain prestigious cooks and chefs publicly scorn the idea of not using and eating quantities of butter, thus sanctioning and abetting others to heap it on thickly. Such attitudes, in the face of evidence that cardiovascular disease is our nation's number one cause of death, are at best a denial and at worst irresponsible.

If there was no concern about personal appearance and weight, perhaps our consumption of unhealthy foods would be much greater than it is. Unfortunately, however, we cannot see the buildup of interior fat or the plaque in our arteries, and so the possibility that the foods we eat may be causing us harm can easily be denied and ignored. Out of sight, out of mind.

The argument is sometimes made that since it took fifty to sixty years to build up the plaque that clogged our arteries and caused the heart attack, our new bypasses have given us many trouble-free years ahead no matter what we eat and whether or not we exercise. This argument is specious. The arteries and veins used in the bypass procedure are out of place in the natural functioning of the body. As such, they are particularly vulnerable to malfunction and disorder. Plaque can quickly build up in them, perhaps more rapidly than in the natural coronary arteries. This might occur simply from the trauma of the surgery itself. A not inconsiderable proportion of these grafts become clogged in a relatively short period of time following surgery. In sum, these bypass grafts need to be treated with extra tender loving care rather than with an attitude of neglect or business as usual. To provide such care, life-affirming habits are called for: eating right, exercising, reducing life stresses, and handling them more effectively (see Chapter 5).

Living As a Cardiac Cripple

A second choice open to the bypass graduate is to become a so-called cardiac cripple. There is potential psychological gain in being an invalid. You may receive the attention and concern from significant others that may have been missing or insufficient in the past. Being an invalid may fulfill unconscious needs for nurturance or dependency and thus, for some individuals, may be rewarding even though, objectively, they have considerable reserves and capacities for autonomous functioning.

One of the common responses of friends and colleagues to my surgery was overconcern about my capacity to work, to be involved socially, and to otherwise live my life normally. I was being treated as if I were an invalid. On one occasion, after a day spent on a long, moderately strenuous hike in my neighborhood, we had dinner at a friend's house. When we drove up to their home, our friend rushed out and pointed to a space in their carport that had been readied for us so that I would not have to walk more than five steps to reach the front door. It was amusing given the strenuous walking I had already done that same day. But, it is not an uncommon occurrence in the lives of bypass graduates after surgery.

Many people think that the surgery leaves the person spent, frail, and crippled, his or her health precarious; the person is often treated as if he or she were going to drop dead any second. This appears to be a common problem faced by bypass graduates. Some male bypass graduates report that their wives do not allow them to work. In one case, the wife sold the husband's business while he was recuperating from bypass surgery, forcing him into what might be a premature retirement. Some spouses of bypass patients are frightened by the experience and want to hold on to and preserve their relationship. The fantasy is that if they treat the mate like an invalid, somehow his or her life will be prolonged.

Surgeons and cardiologists may also unwittingly play a role in promoting cardiac crippling. Some may be good at treating disease, but may not know how to promote health. How physicians encourage their patients to increase their health-promoting behaviors may make the difference between holding on to or giving up their view of themselves as cripples. For example, my experience is that most cardiologists want you to eat the right foods and to exercise. But they often discuss these behaviors— really life-changing activities with little enthusiasm or deep interest in the individual's struggle to make life changes. Saying, "I'd like you to enroll in a rehab program" isn't saying much. It doesn't give the patient an idea of how much this will matter, what a difference it can make. It doesn't deal with the patient's fears or resistance to exercise in the past, or explain the benefits the patient might derive from such a program.

Many of the persons enrolled in rehab programs do not even have an idea of why they are there and believe that once the program is over they can return to their old ways of living. Less than half of the enrollees in the initial postsurgical phase (Phase II) of cardiac rehab programs continue on to more advanced phases. Medicare and some insurance companies will reimburse or pay only for Phase II programs and so only the strongly motivated person would want to proceed onward to a Phase III program, which would incur out-of-pocket expenses.

Of course, one might exercise on one's own, for example, by walking a given distance or for a given amount of time each day. However, this requires self-discipline to compensate for the social support and camaraderie one obtains in group exercise.

Looking Forward

Lastly, you can respond to bypass surgery by seizing the opportunities it presents for renewing your commitment to life. For many, the experience of CAD and bypass surgery is a major turning point in their lives, leading to a reorganization and restructing of almost every aspect of the way they live. Above all, it is a recognition that they cannot go backward to what once was; they can no longer afford the sedentary life of the past, with its denials, lack of consciousness, and self-delusions.

Many bypass graduates feel that they have obtained a reprieve from death—that they have received a warning and have been given a second chance to finish the work that they were born to accomplish. Many have lost their fear of life.

Some individuals emerge from bypass surgery resentful and bitter that this "insult" to their bodily integrity and inner peace has occurred. Some rage that it is unfair, given how well they have taken care of themselves, and actively strive to undo this insult as quickly as possible. Undoing the injury can have positive effects if it leads you to change the self-destructive be-havior of the past. But if it leads to a return to all the habits of the past, then what was it all for? You could have gone on without the surgery, taken your chances in the heart attack lottery, and given lip service to a change in lifestyle.

Bypass surgery can be thought of as a gift. Without it, many of us would either be living as invalids or not be here at all. Because of biomedical advances and the technical skill of a handful of surgeons, bypass surgery gives an increasing number of persons the possibility to live more active, meaningful, and, yes, longer lives. In this sense it is a gift, one that should be treasured and cared for. You care for this particular gift by finding new pur-pose and meaning in your life and your relationships and health-maintaining and -affirming activities.

The decision to have bypass surgery can be accompanied by resolve about many aspects of your life. One of the reasons I advocate psychological preparation for the surgery is that it pro-motes effective healing and renewed dedication to life afterward. Preparing for the surgery requires a commitment to life that in turn promotes a commitment to maintaining the gains achieved by surgery.

One way of making the experience, with all its anxiety and pain, into something meaningful and worthwhile for yourself and your family is to maintain what you gain from the surgery for as long as possible. This can be done by living a healthful life, one in which the factors contributing to CAD are reduced, if not eliminated. A healthful life requires eating the right foods (pref-erably no fat), exercise, management of daily stresses, and adopt-ing the life-affirming attitudes and behavior discussed in the previous chapters.

THE OPENED HEART

My medical colleagues talk about the "plumbing" in my heart having been corrected. But it's not that simple. On the level of feelings, there's a sense that I'm no longer the same. I like to think that I have been reborn and have a second go at life. *Everything* feels so changed, not just a few pipes feeding my heart muscle. I imagine that individuals who have had a heart attack and obligatory bypass surgery feel this even more strongly than I do.

Some individuals experience the lack of "sameness" as a loss of some halcyon past. They yearn to return to the past, but this also requires a return to denial. Denial is one of the major ways humans deal with their fears. Small children, like ostriches, sometimes pretend that if they close their eyes and bury their heads, the big bad wolf doesn't exist. We tolerate such coping behavior in children and even think it's cute. But in adults, such behavior may be self-destructive. It certainly isn't cute.

President Franklin Roosevelt was correct when he said, "The only thing we have to fear is fear itself." Fear of growing old, of death, of making fools of ourselves, etc., leads us to do some rather positive things such as taking care of our health, being superprepared for a public speech, etc. Fear, however, may alternatively lead to denial that we will ever make fools of ourselves, or grow old, or die. Growing in the soil of fear, such denials may lead us to believe we are immune to human faults and natural events. "They will not happen to me." This delusion may acquire enormous force in our lives and direct our attitudes, behavior, and feelings along very destructive lines. This is particularly true when it comes to the maintenance of our bodies and our health.

Fear keeps us from acknowledging that life has its limits. We will not live forever. We will not experience everything there is to experience. We will not see everything and do everything there is to do. In short, living one's life effectively without fear means accepting the reality that there are limits and that being human means having limitations. If one cannot accept that life has limitations, then one may have difficulty accepting that life has to change after bypass surgery.

Bypass surgery brings us face to face with fear. It is an opportunity to face our fears with honesty and to let go of the denials, delusions, and lies we tell ourselves about our lives. Bypass surgery is an opportunity to master our fears about life. Such mastery comes from the conscious choices we make about our lives and from our responses to the new opportunities second chances bring.

One of the major opportunities available at this time is to get in touch with the deep inner well of emotional resources that bypass surgery inevitably unseals and liberates. The heart is literally and figuratively opened up to love, tenderness, compassion, forgiveness; to things of beauty—simple, basic things that warm us from within, make us feel closer to others and part of the flow of creation, and that bathe us with an inestimable sense of goodness and aliveness. Tears come to our eyes as we reconnect with sensations, sights, sounds, and smells sometimes associated with tender memories from a simpler, pristine past, reminding us how deeply we are able to feel and comprehend the essentials of life.

The opened heart is a treasure that the trauma of heart attack or bypass surgery makes available to us, reminding us of our fragility and finiteness and the extent to which our feelings and emotions have been dulled by daily events. It reminds us, too, of how much we need to be with and to cherish others and to be cherished by them in turn. These reminders bring us in touch with what is really important in the cosmos. How foolish can we be to believe that our tears represent depression or something to be shunned?

Our hearts are our emotional as well as our vascular centers. Thus, in addition to the medical implications, opening and exposing this organ can be experienced as a profound emotional event that allows feelings both to flow forth and to enter. The fact that in the immediate postsurgical period the walls of our usual psychological defenses are down permits the gates of emotion to stand open so that feelings both emanate from and reach our core self. For individuals who have chronically closed their hearts to feelings, the postsurgical period may provide a reawakening, perhaps frightening for some. But this fear, like others, can be confronted and conquered, leaving the person enriched and with a deeper, more intense ability to give and receive love.

We have understood for millennia that the heart is the center and place of origin of our feelings of love. The opened heart allows our feelings of love to touch others and us be touched by them in turn. How sad it is that so many of us need this awesome surgery to revive our connection to this core part of our emotional life. To let this newly opened and rekindled emotional flame fade from disuse because of fear would be an opportunity missed and squandered.

SUGGESTED READING

Frank, A. W. 1991. *At the Will of the Body*. Boston: Houghton Mifflin Co.

Frankl, V. E. 1984. *Man's Search for Meaning*. New York: Washington Square Press.

INDEX

. . . .